Nicole E. Steidle

Micro- and Nanostructured Microfluidic Devices for Localized Protein Immobilization and Other Biomedical Applications

Schriften des Instituts für Mikrostrukturtechnik
am Karlsruher Institut für Technologie (KIT)
Band 29

Hrsg. Institut für Mikrostrukturtechnik

Eine Übersicht aller bisher in dieser Schriftenreihe
erschienenen Bände finden Sie am Ende des Buchs.

Micro- and Nanostructured Microfluidic Devices for Localized Protein Immobilization and Other Biomedical Applications

by
Nicole E. Steidle

KIT Scientific Publishing

Dissertation, Karlsruher Institut für Technologie (KIT)
Fakultät für Maschinenbau

Tag der mündlichen Prüfung: 24. Juni 2014
Hauptreferent: Prof. Dr. Andreas E. Guber
Korreferent: Prof. Dr. Volker Saile, Prof. Dr. Petra S. Dittrich

Impressum

KIT Scientific Publishing

Karlsruher Institut für Technologie (KIT)
KIT Scientific Publishing
Straße am Forum 2
D-76131 Karlsruhe

KIT Scientific Publishing is a registered trademark of Karlsruhe Institute of Technology. Reprint using the book cover is not allowed.

www.ksp.kit.edu

Print on Demand 2015

ISSN 1869-5183
ISBN 978-3-7315-0297-5
DOI 10.5445/KSP/1000044095

Karlsruhe Institute of Technology

Micro- and Nanostructured Microfluidic Devices for Localized Protein Immobilization and Other Biomedical Applications

Zur Erlangung des akademischen Grades
Doktor der Ingenieurswissenschaften
der Fakultät für Maschinenbau des
Karlsruher Instituts für Technologie (KIT)

genehmigte **Dissertation**
von

Dipl.-Ing. Nicole E. Steidle

Tag der mündlichen Prüfung: 24. Juni 2014
Hauptreferent: Prof. Dr. Andreas E. Guber (KIT)
Korreferenten: Prof. Dr. Volker Saile (KIT)
Prof. Dr. Petra S. Dittrich (ETH Zürich)

Abstract

Microfluidics has been a growing field for the last 30 years. Especially, the wide variety of applications in medicine and biology render it more and more interesting. So called Lab-on-a-Chip devices integrate different processes which are used in a laboratory for example to analyze blood samples, on one single chip. This leads to faster analysis, low analyte volumes and the possibility of point-of-care diagnostics. To achieve an inexpensive manufacturing, polymeric materials are of great interest. However, these materials lead to an unspecific adsorption of biomolecules on their surfaces, due to the hydrophilic characteristics of most polymers.

In this work a new immobilization method is introduced for the localized adsorption of proteins on thermoplastic surfaces. Artificial three-phase interfaces were realized by controlling the wetting behavior of the surface which in turn lead to a preferred adsorption in these areas. Afterwards, different fabrication methods were analyzed to determine the mass fabrication capabilities of the proposed design. By combining hot embossing and microthermoforming the fabrication of completely structured microchannels was possible. This method was additionally used to fabricate tubes and micropipettes with structures on the inside and outside. Fully structured channels were examined by contact angle measurements and micro particle image velocimetry to gain information about the influence of the micro- and nanostructures on fluid behavior. The use of injection molding for the fabrication of the proposed immobilization design was also discussed. The design functionality was then examined by protein adsorption experiments, showing a localized adsorption on structured areas for bovine serum albumin (BSA) and streptavidin. These experiments were followed by sandwich-assays for the detection of c-reactive protein in buffer solution as well as in human serum. For both sets of experiments a clear distinction between different concentrations could be made. At the end, cell experiments were conducted on different polymeric materials with micro- and nanostructures, showing a good biocompatibility. After the analysis of the cell growth on differently structured surfaces, new designs were proposed for continuing cell experiments.

The proposed immobilization method enables the use of thermoplastic materials for biological and medical experiments. Additionally, the design is fully capable of mass fabrication by hot embossing, microthermoforming or injection molding. The gained information about fluid behavior as well as cell behavior enable the fabrication and design of devices adapted to an application.

Kurzfassung

Die Mikrofluidik beschäftigt sich mit der Handhabung von kleinen Flüssigkeitsmengen in Mikrokanälen. Dieses Gebiet hat in den letzten 30 Jahren immer mehr an Bedeutung gewonnen. Besonders die Vielzahl an Anwendungen in der Biologie und Medizin machen es besonders interessant. In sogenannten Lab-on-a-Chip Systemen können Prozesse zur Analyse von z.B. Blutproben in einem mikrofluidischen Chip abgebildet werden. Dies führt zu kürzeren Analysezeiten, geringeren Analytvolumina und der Möglichkeit, die Analyse direkt vor Ort durchzuführen (Point-of-Care POC Diagnostics). Um eine kostengünstige Fertigung zu ermöglichen sind besonders Kunststoffe von großer Bedeutung. Jedoch führen Kunststoffoberflächen, aufgrund ihrer hydrophilen Eigenschaft, zu einer unspezifischen Adsorption von Biomolekülen auf der gesamten Oberfläche.

In dieser Arbeit wurde ein neues Immobilisationsverfahren zur lokalisierten Adsorption von Proteinen entwickelt. Dazu wurden künstliche drei-Phasengrenzen an Mikro- und Nanostrukturen erzeugt um eine bevorzugte Adsorption an diesen Stellen zu erreichen. Anschließend wurde das vorgestellte Design auf seine Massenfertigungstauglichkeit geprüft. Dabei wurden verschiedene Verfahren zur Herstellung verwendet, wie z.B. Heißprägen und Mikrothermoformen. Durch die Kombination von Heißprägen und Mikrothermoformen sowie eines Bondverfahrens, wie z.B. Laserschweißens, konnte eine Vielzahl von strukturierten dreidimensionalen Bauteilen hergestellt werden. In dieser Arbeit wurden Mikroschläuche, Mikropipetten und mikrofluidische Kanalstrukturen hergestellt und charakterisiert. Dazu wurden Kontaktwinkelmessungen sowie Particel Tracking Velocimetry verwendet. Zusätzlich wurde auch die Herstellung mittels Spritzgießen bzw. Spritzprägen für das vorgestellte Immobilisierungsverfahren diskutiert. Im Anschluss wurde das Immobilisationsverfahren für Rinderserumalbumin (BSA) sowie Streptavidin getestet. Dabei konnte die Funktionsweise des Verfahrens validiert werden. Um das Verfahren noch in einem realen Anwendungsfall zu testen, wurden Immunoassays (Sandwich-Assays) zur Detektion von c-reaktiven Protein in Pufferlösung und in Serum durchgeführt. Dabei konnten in Pufferlösung sowie in Serum unterschiedliche Konzentrationen des c-reaktiven Proteins nachgewiesen werden. Abschließend wurden erste Zellversuche durchgeführt, wobei eine sehr gute Biokompatibilität von verschiedenen Kunststoffen nachgewiesen werden konnte. Nach Untersuchung des Zellverhaltens auf unterschiedlich strukturierten Oberflächen wurden weitere Designs erstellt führ weiterführende Zellversuche.

Das vorgestellte Immobilisierungsverfahren ermöglicht die Verwendung von Kunststoffen ohne zeitaufwendige Nachbearbeitung und Oberflächenmodifikationen. Verschiedene industriellen Standardverfahren können zur Herstellung verwendet werden. Die Hergestellten Diagnose-Chips haben sich zusätzlich durch eine hohe Robustheit sowie einfach Handhabung ausgezeichnet. Dies sind wichtige Voraussetzungen für ein Lab-on-a-Chip System für die Point-of-Care Diagnostik.

Acknowledgment

Working in science is never fruitful in solitary. Many people influence ones work with discussions and ideas. Following, I want to say my gratitude to some of these people who helped me realize my ideas and supported me in this work.

My gratitude goes to Prof. Dr. Andreas E. Guber. He gave me the opportunity to conduct research at the Institute of Microstructure Technology (IMT) at the Karlsruhe Institute of Technology. He also supervised my work and ensured optimal working conditions. I also want to thank Prof. Dr. Volker Saile, who inspired me to work in the field of microtechnology.

Furthermore, it is a pleasure to acknowledge Prof. Dr. Petra S. Dittrich (ETH Zürich), for the fruitful discussions and the opportunity to take a peek into Biology at her lab. I am indepted to Felix Kurth and Klaus Eyer for conducting the cell experiments and explaining me the details of cell culturing. Thank you, Dr. Tom Robinson for your time in capturing images at the confocal laser scanning microscope. At this point, I want to acknowledge the financial support from the Karlsruhe House of Young Scientist (KHYS) for my research visit at the ETH-Zürich, as well as for various workshops and trainings.

I am very much indebted to Bürkert Fluid Control Systems GmbH, for the financial support but also for the supervision of my work and many discussions. Especially, I want to thank Dr. Thomas Hahn for co-supervising my work, Dr. Raoul Schröder for being my contact person in all matters that arrived, and Dr. Dieter Binz for welcoming me so warmly in his Research and Development group.

Without the help of many colleagues at the IMT this work would not have been possible. I want to thank the team of Alexandra Moritz, for fabricating all requested parts with the greatest precision. For the numerous tries of fabricating mold inserts by direct laser writing, my gratitude goes to Stefan Hengsbach. Paul Abbaffy spent many hours at the scanning electron microscopy to achieve great SEM micrographs. For his great passion of catching the essence of a sample, I want to thank him. I also thank the Karlsruhe Nano Micro Facilities (KNMF) for giving me access to the necessary equipment.

I especially want to thank Dr. Ralf Ahrens. He spent numerous hours proof-reading my manuscript as well as my publications. I also want to thank my office mate Felix Marschall for his friendship and support.

I am indebted to my cooperation partners at the Institute of Fluid Mechanics, especially Prof. Dr. Bettina Frohnapfel and Dr. Jochen Kriegseis, for many discussions and input to my work.

My thanks also go to my students, Anja Lepple, Ali El-Zein, Nefta Kanilmaz, Ellen Bengtson, Elena Rubiu, Christian Bader, Patrick Tritschler, Gerlinde Utsch and Paulina Monard, for their laborious work and support.

My greatest thank you goes to Marc Schneider, Dr. Alexander Kolew and PD Dr. Matthias Worgull. Their deep knowledge of fabrication methods enabled the great results achieved in this work.

For many fruitful discussions I want to thank: Dr. Bastian Rapp, Dr. Michael Röhrig, Dr. Kerstin Länge, Dr. Friederike Gruhl, Richard Thelen, Christian Lay, Dr. Arndt Last, Dr. Danays Kunka, Dr. Sebastian Köber, Norbert Schneider, Dr. Markus Simon, Dr. Maryna Kavalenka, Radwanul Siddique and Dr. Jacques Fattaccioli.

Finally, I would like to give my gratitude to my family and to my husband Tobias, for their love and support.

Karlsruhe, May 2014 *Nicole E. Steidle*

Contents

Abstract . . . . **i**

Kurzfassung . . . . **iii**

Acknowledgment . . . . **v**

1 Introduction **1**

2 Theory and Design Development **5**

2.1 Basic Principles of Proteins 5

2.1.1 Protein Structure 5

2.1.2 Protein - Surface Interactions 6

2.1.3 Proteins and Interfaces 8

2.2 Wetting Behavior 10

2.3 State of the Art of Protein Immobilization 14

2.4 Design Development 15

2.4.1 Factors of Influence 16

2.4.2 Design Parameters 17

3 Fabrication Processes for Structured Microfluidic Devices **21**

3.1 Basic Principles 23

3.1.1 Materials 24

3.1.2 Mold fabrication 25

3.2 Hot Embossing 27

3.2.1 Experimental 29

3.2.2 Modification A: Double sided hot embossing 33

3.2.3 Modification B: Hot Pulling 34
3.2.4 Mold Insert Fabrication 37
3.3 Microthermoforming 38
3.3.1 Experimental 39
3.3.2 Modification A: Thermoformbonding 41
3.3.3 Modification B: Twin-Sheet-Forming 43
3.4 Bonding 45
3.4.1 Adhesive Bonding 45
3.4.2 Thermobonding 46
3.4.3 Laser Welding 46
3.5 Injection Molding 47
3.6 Discussion and Outlook 50

4 Properties and Applications of Structured Microfluidic Devices 51
4.1 Measurement of the Wetting Behavior 51
4.1.1 Experimental Setup 51
4.1.2 Results and Discussion 53
4.2 Dynamic Fluid Behavior 56
4.2.1 Theory and State of the Art 56
4.2.2 Experimental Setup 60
4.2.3 Results 62
4.3 Further Applications in Medicine 66
4.3.1 Tubes 67
4.3.2 Micropipette 69
4.4 Conclusion and Outlook 69

5 Proteinadsorption 73
5.1 Laser Scanning and Fluorescence Microscopy 74
5.2 Localized Protein Immobilization 75
5.2.1 Experimental Setup 75
5.2.2 Results 77

5.3 Sandwich-Assays 86
5.3.1 State of the Art 87
5.3.2 Experimental Setup 88
5.3.3 Results 92
5.4 Conclusion 95

6 Cell Experiments 99
6.1 Basic Principles 100
6.1.1 Cells 100
6.1.2 Cell Culture Substrates 101
6.1.3 Sterilization 101
6.2 Experimental Setup 103
6.3 Results and Discussion 104
6.4 Conclusion and Outlook 107

7 Conclusion and Outlook 109

A List of Publications 113
A.1 Patents 113
A.2 Articles 113
A.3 Conference Contributions 114
A.4 Seminar Talks at other Institutes 115

Bibliography 138

1. Introduction

Since the visionary talk of Richard P. Feynman[1] in 1959, miniaturization has entered every part of our life, from nanometer transistors on CPUs to miniaturized cameras and acceleration sensors in cell phones. Even single atom manipulation is already possible.[2] Now microscopy technologies enable the visualization of surfaces at nanoscopic dimensions, mankind can see the micro- and nanotechnologies nature has been using for millennia. One famous example is the lotus leaf,[3] which can self-clean due to the micro- and nanostructures on its surface. Nature shows us even more applications, like the water harvesting of the Stenocara beetle in the Namib Desert,[4] the friction reduction of shark skin[5] and the colors of butterfly wings.[6]

Also in medicine and biology miniaturized systems are gaining more and more influence. For example, tools with only a few hundred micrometers in dimension are utilized for minimal invasive surgery.[7] Also for diagnostic purposes and drug screening, miniaturized fluidic systems are essential.[8,9] These so called Lab-on-a-Chip (LOC) or micro Total Analyis Systems (μTAS) enable fast processing of small analyte volumes, as well as the possibility of hand-held devices and, therefore, Point-of-Care diagnostics. Today Lab-on-a-Chip devices find numerous applications starting with fundamental research like cell studies[10,11] to full diagnostic devices.[12] However, these devices are still not established in the market. One current limitation is their expensive and laborious fabrication process. Often many different process steps are necessary to fabricate microfluidic devices.[13] Additionally, point-of-care diagnostic is still in its infancy because of a missing miniaturization of read-out devices.

The aim of this work was to develop a new protein immobilization method to enable an inexpensive mass fabrication capable Lab-on-a-Chip system. To achieve this, micro- and nanostructured thermoplastic polymers are utilized. These structures can also influence the wetting behavior, friction as well as cell growth. All of which this work will address.

The proposed immobilization method utilizes a protein transport mechanism to interfaces. By fabricating artificial three-phase interfaces on thermoplastic polymeric materials, a preferred adsorption of proteins on desired locations within a microfluidic channel is shown to be possible. Here in, first design parameters are discussed to fabricate superhydrophobic surfaces in the Cassie-Baxter state. This state is characterized by trapped air between micro- or nanostructures on the surfaces. Therefore, a liquid-gas-solid interface is achieved. This interface leads to a protein transport and a higher protein adsorption in these areas. Theory, parameters and experiments are discussed in Chapter 2.

After the development of a new detection protocol and fluid control possibilities different fabrication methods are examined. Chapter 3 investigates methods capable of mass fabrication to bring the proposed microfluidic device closer to market. For fully structured microfluidic channels a combination of hot embossing, microthermoforming and laser welding is utilized. This is compared to a combination of hot embossing and injection molding as a fabrication method for microfluidic diagnostic devices.

Chapter 4 deals with fluidic properties in fully structured microfluidic channels. First, contact angle measurements are conducted to gain information about the influence of structure dimensions and material on the wetting behavior. Afterwards, micro astigmatism particle tracking velocimetry sheds light on velocity profiles inside structured channels. This chapter also discusses the application of micro- and nanostructured tubes for medical equipment like venous catheters.

Afterwards, the proposed chip design is used for protein adsorption experiments. These experiments examine the adsorption on micro- and nanostructured surfaces in the Cassie-Baxter state. Furthermore, this Lab-on-a-Chip system is used to detect a typical protein, produced by the body in case of an inflammation, in buffer solution as well as in human serum, and will show the potential of this new method (see Chapter 5).

During a research visit and collaboration at the ETH Zürich, first cell experiments with differently structured surfaces are conducted. These cell experiments are summarized in Chapter 6. New design parameters as well as possibilities for further experiments and applications in tissue engineering and for cell growth experiments are given. The work ends with a summary and outlook (Chapter 7).

2. Theory and Design Development

In this chapter, basic principles of proteins are introduced. Different protein-surface interactions are explained as well as factors influencing the protein adsorption, leading to a preferred movement of proteins towards interfaces. This accumulation of proteins onto interfaces lead to the idea of a localized protein immobilization on artificial interfaces. To achieve such interfaces, the wetting behavior of a surface has to be controlled. Hence, the second part of this chapter covers the wetting behavior of fluids on surfaces. At the end of this chapter, a new design is introduced to immobilize proteins on surfaces without any laborious surface treatments.

2.1. Basic Principles of Proteins

2.1.1. Protein Structure

Proteins are assembled from amino acids, which are joined covalently by dehydration. If more then 50 amino acids are linked together, the amino acid chain is defined as a protein, less linked amino acids are known as polypeptides. The function of a protein is determined by the contained amino acids and its sequence.[14,15]

Proteins have a three dimensional structure with a favored structure, leading to a minimum free enthalpy. In this structure, called native conformation, the biological functions can be performed. The primary structure of a protein is its sequence of amino acids. This molecular backbone in a selected segment is spatially arranged in the secondary structure. To complete the three-dimensional structure of a protein, the secondary structures are again arranged in a tertiary structure. Two kinds of tertiary structures are known, fibrous and globular. The fibrous proteins have simple repeating elements of secondary structures, while globular proteins contain several types of secondary structures of the same polypeptide chain. The last structure, the quaternary structure, describes the arrangement of larger proteins composed of different domains or of small globular proteins linked together.[14,16]

2.1.2. Protein - Surface Interactions

The complex structure of proteins leads to an inhomogeneous surface of the protein with domains of different characteristics (see Figure 2.1) which, in turn, lead to different protein-surface interactions depending on the protein orientation towards the surface. Covalent bonds and additionally five general classes of non-covalent forces and interactions are important for proteins:[16]

- Van-der-Waals interactions
- Electrostatic interactions
- Hydrogen bonding
- Hydrophobic interactions
- Other interactions, like charge-transfer or $\pi - \pi$ interactions.

Covalent Immobilization

A covalent bond is present, when two atoms share two electrons between them. These shared electrons lead to a stable electron configuration, because the atoms have enough electrons to fill their outer shell and therefore are in an energetic favorable state. Additionally, the negative charge of the electrons counteracts the positive charge of the atom nucleus and leads to a closer packing. This bond is directional and will determine the three

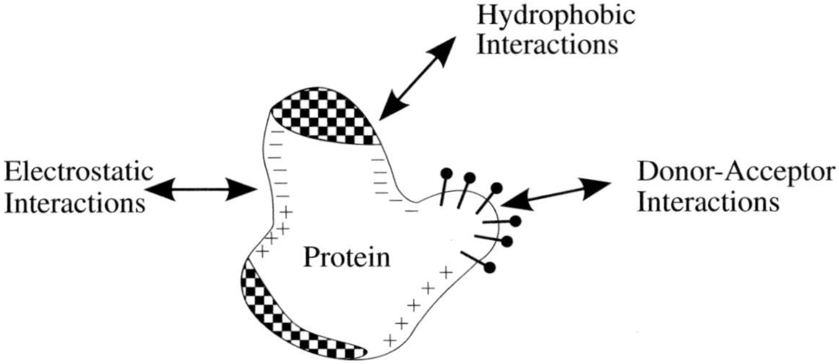

Figure 2.1.: Schematic view of a protein with different domains, leading to different interactions with the surface depending on the orientation during approach. (modified after Andrade *et al.*[16])

dimensional structure. Covalent forces, like almost all intermolecular interactions, decrease with an increase of distance.[14,15,17]

Non-covalent Immobilization

As biomolecules carry a large number of charged groups, electrostatic interactions are of great importance. The electrostatic interactions are governed by the Coulomb law describing the interaction of two point charges in vacuum. This force is inversely proportional to the square of the distance $F_c \propto \frac{1}{r^2}$. Electrostatic forces are also weakened by two effects, commonly found in biological and medical experiments. Biomolecules are solubilized in a buffer solution, often with a high salt concentration, leading to free ions shielding the charged surfaces. Additionally, water, with its high dipole moment, and therefore high dielectric constant is amplifying this shielding effect. Both effects lead to an decrease of the range of the electrostatic forces.[15,17]

Hydrogen bonding is a special case of dipole-dipole interaction and is achieved when a positive charged hydrogen interacts with two free electron pairs. These interactions are normally very weak. But due to the small size and large dipole moment of water, strong attractive forces can be achieved.

Especially strong bonds are known for hydrogen with nitrogen, oxygen, sulfur and fluorine.[15,17]

Based on the ability of water to form hydrogen bonds, hydrophobic interactions play an important role between non-polar molecules in water. One water molecule can participate in four hydrogen bonds, acting as a proton donor and as a proton acceptor twice for each case. But in contact with a non-polar molecule, hydrogen bonds are not possible, therefore the water molecules order around these areas, called hydrophobic areas. The non-polar molecules in contrast will also try to decrease the contact between hydrophobic areas and water. This leads to a clustering of hydrophobic regions and is called hydrophobic interaction. The strength of the hydrophobic interaction is a direct result of the system achieving thermodynamic stability. Additionally, the clustering of hydrophobic areas of proteins gives the protein more stability.[14,17,15]

Adsorption of biomolecules is a well studied but complicated phenomenon.[18] A multitude of interactions play a role in the adsorption process, especially electrostatic and hydrophobic interactions. To make matters worse, proteins can also change their conformation when in contact with a liquid or solid, leading to a change of characteristics.[18]

2.1.3. Proteins and Interfaces

Adsorption deals in general with the accumulation of a substance at an interface.[19] In solution the adsorption on a surface is an exchange process, because the adsorbing molecule is replacing a solvent molecule and the adsorbing molecule partly leaves the solvent environment. The adsorption rate increases meanwhile for hydrophobic molecules, because they are repelled by the water.

Norde und Lyklema[20] described the preferred adsorption of proteins on interfaces. They determined three factors leading to a higher accumulation of proteins at interfaces (between solid, liquid or gas). The first factor is the dehydration of parts of the surface and of protein molecules. Dehydration describes the loss of a water molecule from the reacting molecule and leads to a decrease in the Gibbs energy of the system. This in turn is followed by a favored adsorption in these areas. The Gibbs energy G (Eq. 2.1) is described by the enthalpy H, entropy S and temperature T. $\triangle_{ads}$ describes meanwhile the change of the function due to adsorption processes.

$$\triangle_{ads} G = \triangle_{ads} H - T \cdot \triangle_{ads} S < 0 \tag{2.1}$$

Adsorption is favored for a decrease in Gibbs energy, which can be induced by an increase in temperature, increase in entropy or a decrease in enthalpy. An increase in temperature additionally increases the diffusion rate and leads also to higher protein adsorption.[21] The large contribution of the protein to the dehydration of a hydrophobic sorbent leads to the adsorption of proteins on any surface with hydrophobic domains.[20] This process takes even place under unfavorable electrostatic conditions.

The second influence factor is a redistribution of charged groups due to overlapping of the electrical double layer. A surface in contact with a fluid is charged by either ionization or dissociation of surface groups or by adsorption of ions.[17] Counterions will order around the surface, leading to a potential between surface and the layer of counterions. This layer is called the outer Helmholtz layer and is followed by a diffuse layer of ions in motion, called the stern layer. The electrical double layer leads to an electrokinetic potential between the surface and any molecule in the liquid. This in turn induces electrical forces and a motion of charged particles.

When proteins move from an aqueous solution to an interface the change of environment can also lead to a rearrangement of the protein structure. The three-dimensional structure is highly dependent on the environment. For example, hydrophobic domains will be placed inside the protein, avoiding contact with the aqueous solution. The structure is therefore stabilized by hydrophobic interactions. In close proximity to a surface, other interactions favoring an expanded structure could lead to a structural change of the protein. This occurs when hydrophobic domains are in contact with a surface, while still avoiding contact with the aqueous solution. By rearranging the protein structure the entropy is increasing, emphasizing adsorption due to a decrease in the Gibbs energy.

In general, proteins tend to adsorb more readily on non-polar, charged surfaces with high surface tensions.[21]

2.2. Wetting Behavior

The wetting behavior describes the properties of a liquid in contact with a solid surface. In general, this is examined by placing a liquid droplet on the surface. This droplet either spreads over the surface or forms a spherical shape. This leads to a triple line at the solid-liquid-gas interface. The angle between the surface and the liquid at the triple line is defined as the contact angle and is used to classify surfaces. Traditionally four groups are known as shown in Table 2.1.[22]

Table 2.1.: Classification of surfaces by their contact angle Θ_0.

$\Theta_0 \leq 10°$	$10° < \Theta_0 < 90°$	$90° < \Theta_0 \leq 150°$	$\Theta_0 > 150°$
supderhydrophilic	hydrophilic	hydrophobic	superhydrophobic

Surfaces with contact angles below 90° are called hydrophilic, which can be translated into water loving. Most polymeric materials have hydrophilic surface properties in their natural state. Contact angles over 90° are generally describing hydrophobic, water repellent, surfaces. These surfaces are well studied because of their wide occurrence in nature. When taking a closer look at the most famous representative, the lotus leaf, superhydrophobic surfaces can lead to a self-cleaning effect of the surface.[3] In this particular example the measured contact angles of the lotus leaves are very high and at the same time display a low adhesion. The adhesion can be described by the contact angle hysteresis, which is the difference between advancing Θ_{adv} and receding Θ_{rec} contact angle. A schematic view of the contact angle hysteresis is shown in Figure 2.2. Low contact angle hystereses lead to a movement of the liquid droplet at slightly inclined surfaces. High contact angle hystereses are often observed, when surface defects lead to a pinning of the droplet or the surface roughness leads to a high adhesion. This effects can lead to a wide range of measured contact angles for one surface. Thereby, the advancing and receding contact angles define the range of possible contact angles on a surface.

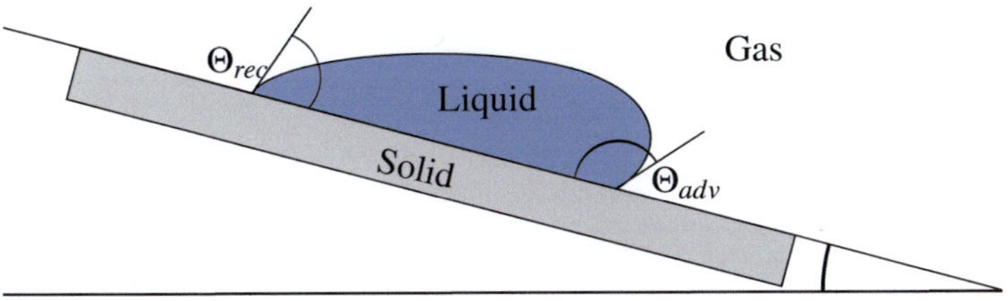

Figure 2.2.: Schematic depiction of the Contact Angle Hysteresis.

The wetting of surfaces can be described by different theoretical models. The basis for all models is the Young equation (Eq. 2.2) formulated by T. Young in 1805.[23] This equation describes the contact angle as a force balance between three interfaces at the contact line. When arguing on a molecular scale, a water molecule inside a droplet feels intermolecular forces evenly distributed to all sides. A molecule on the boundary will feel forces primarily to the inside of the droplet. Therefore, work has to be done when moving a water molecule to the interface.[19] This work is defined as the specific surface tension. Because additional interactions with the environment are present, interfacial surface tensions γ_{SG}, γ_{LS} and γ_{LG} between the solid-gas, liquid-solid and liquid-gas interfaces, are further used to describe the system. The Young Equation represents the force balance between these three surface tensions.

$$\gamma_{SG} - \gamma_{LS} = \gamma_{LG} \cdot \cos\Theta_0 \tag{2.2}$$

This equation is valid for homogeneous, smooth and ideal surfaces. A schematic depiction of the Young contact angle is given in Figure 2.3.

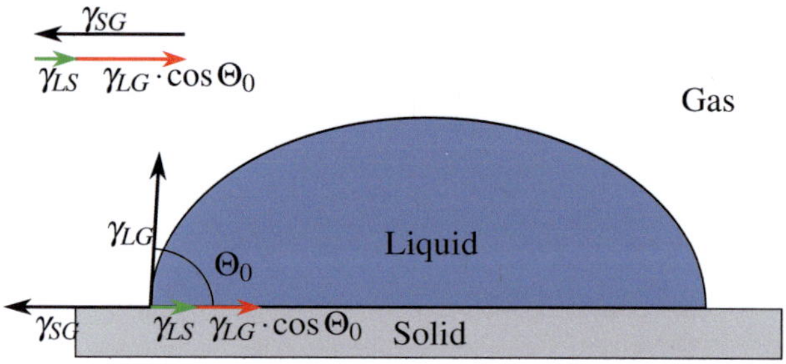

Figure 2.3.: Schematic view of the Young state.

For non-ideal surfaces the Young equation was extended first by Wenzel in 1936[24] and in 1944 by Cassie and Baxter.[25] Both equations take the roughness of the surface into account. Figure 2.4 shows a schematic view of the wetting behavior in the (a) Wenzel state and in the (b) Cassie and Baxter state.

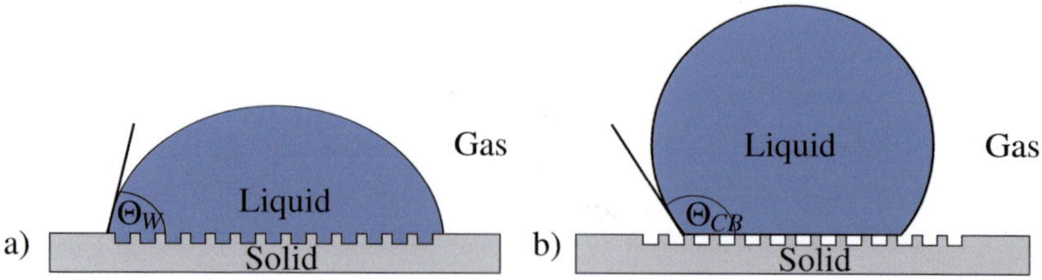

Figure 2.4.: Schematic view of the a) Wenzel state and b) Cassie-Baxter state.

In the Wenzel state a droplet placed on a rough surface will spread over the surface and follow the surface topography. Depending on the roughness of the surface the contact angle will either be increased or decreased. The change of contact angle is proportional to the roughness factor r, which is the ratio of the area of the real surface to the area of the ideal surface (Eq. 2.3) and is always greater 1.

$$r = \frac{A_{real}}{A_{ideal}} > 1 \tag{2.3}$$

$$\cos\Theta_W = r \cdot \cos\Theta_0 \tag{2.4}$$

The roughness factor is extending the Young equation and is taking the real surface area into account. The Wenzel equation (Eq. 2.4) states, that a hydrophilic surface with a contact angle of $\Theta_0 < 90°$ can, by increasing the roughness factor, become more hydrophilic. For materials with contact angles of $\Theta_0 > 90°$ an increase of the roughness factor would in turn lead to an increase of contact angle. The equation also states, that it is not possible to change a hydrophilic material into a hydrophobic material and vice versa by surface structuring. Because the droplet follows the surface topography, the Wenzel state is also characterized by a large contact angle hysteresis,[26] due to pinning effects on the surface structures.

Another description of real surfaces is given by Cassie and Baxter. They argued that a droplet will not penetrate the surface structures but lie on top of the structures, which is also known as the Fakir-State. In the Cassie-Baxter state not only a liquid-solid interface is formed but also a liquid-gas interface. With this the Young equation is extended by the area f_1 of the liquid-solid-interface while the liquid-gas-interface f_2 is subtracted (Eq. 2.5). To obtain a very high contact angle the liquid-solid interface should be as small as possible.

$$\cos\Theta_{CB} = f_1 \cdot \cos\Theta_0 - f_2 \tag{2.5}$$

Depending on the height of the surface structures, the droplet can also be in a metastable Cassie-Baxter state.[26] When the Wenzel state is the less energetic state of the droplet, a carefully placed droplet can be in the Cassie-Baxter state. The droplet in this metastable Cassie-Baxter state can be transition into the Wenzel state with a slight disturbance. This disturbance can be vibration of the substrate, pressure on the droplet or impact on the surface.

Liquids in the Cassie-Baxter state have a lower contact angle hysteresis than droplets in the Wenzel state. This is due to the decreased contact area and therefore less pinning to the surface. Superhydrophobic, self-cleaning surfaces, like the lotus leaf, are known to be in the Cassie-Baxter state.

2.3. State of the Art of Protein Immobilization

Localized protein immobilization has many applications in biology and medicine. Two groups of localized immobilization methods are known: mechanical methods and photo-lithography.

Mechanical methods use physical means, like printing or deposition, to immobilize proteins. Typically microwells are utilized to define areas of protein adsorption or cell growth. To place proteins or cells only inside the wells the area between the wells is either passivated[27] or the wells can be fabricated out of Polyethylen glycol (PEG), which prohibits protein or cell adhesion. After settlement of the cells or proteins inside the PEG-wells, the well plate is washed and molecules outside the wells are washed away. Another method, allowing the patterning of proteins, is micro contact printing. This method was introduced by Bernard *et al.*[28] in 2000. A soft stamp is wetted with a protein solution. Upon conformal contact with a surface the proteins are transferred. Other methods utilize superhydrophilic and superhydrophobic surface characteristics to define areas of protein adsorption.[29] In 1995 a process called MIMIC - micromolding in capillaries - was proposed by Kim *et al.*[30] This method utilizes an elastomeric stamp with capillaries forming a network of channels. This stamp is placed on a substrate and a droplet of liquid pre-polymer is deposited in front of the channel entrance. The liquid polymer is sucked into the capillaries by capillary forces and the polymer can be cross-linked either thermally or photochemically. The used polymer is protein repellent, leading to an adsorption in the unstructured areas.[31,32]

Photo-lithography is either used to change the properties of the surface photochemically or to pattern the proteins directly. When changing the surface properties the protein-surface interactions are controlled leading to protein adsorption or cell growth or a prohibition of it. This method is highly dependent on the material and therefore, only a small number of materials are used with the most common being PEG. A direct patterning of proteins can be done by photo-activateable molecules. These molecules have linked fluorophores, which are excited by light. This excitation leads to photobleaching due to resonance and to a covalent attachment of the fluorophore to BSA.[33] For all photo-lithographic methods different patterning procedures are possible. Most of them use a mask to define the pattern. Others use direct patterning techniques like a laser or, to achieve higher cycle times, combine the laser patterning with a digital mirror device.[34]

2.4. Design Development

After reviewing various articles[31,34,35,36,37] a new method for the localized adsorption of proteins is developed. The basic principle is based on the movement of proteins to interfaces. Therefore, a chip is designed with artificial triple interfaces. This can be achieved by a liquid in the Cassie-Baxter state. In this state air is trapped between surface structures and a three-phase interface is realized between the trapped air, the structures and the liquid on top of the structures. First different factors are discussed to control the Cassie-Baxter state. Afterwards, design parameters are given to fabricate surfaces, which lead to a fluid in the Cassie-Baxter state.

2.4.1. Factors of Influence

When designing structured surfaces leading to a fluid in the Cassie-Baxter state, several factors have to be considered. Shirtcliffe *et al.*[38] examined the influence of the height of the structures on the contact angle. They showed, that for a aspect ratio of greater 1, the maximum contact angle was reached and the fluid was in the Cassie-Baxter state. At a aspect ratio of less than 1 the fluid was in a metastable Cassie-Baxter state or the Wenzel state (see Figure 2.5). This transition can be explained by taking the energy per unit area into account,[26] leading to an energy barrier which is proportionally to the height of the pillars. Also Patankar[39] showed, that the Cassie-Baxter state can be achieved for high aspect ratios.

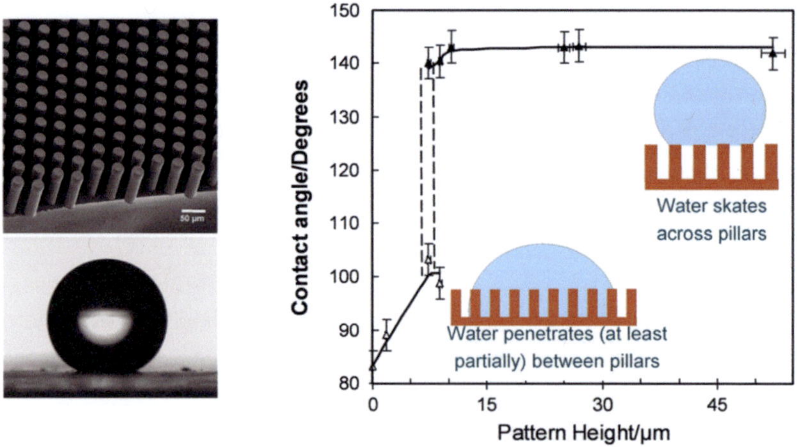

Figure 2.5.: Dependency of the contact angle on the height of a pillar with a diameter of 15 µm.[40]

In 2012 Kashaninejad *et al.*[41] studied the influence of microstructure alignment. It was shown, that by starting from a checkerboard pattern and changing the layout by moving the lines against each other, the contact angle decreases with an increase of the eccentricity (see Figure 2.6).

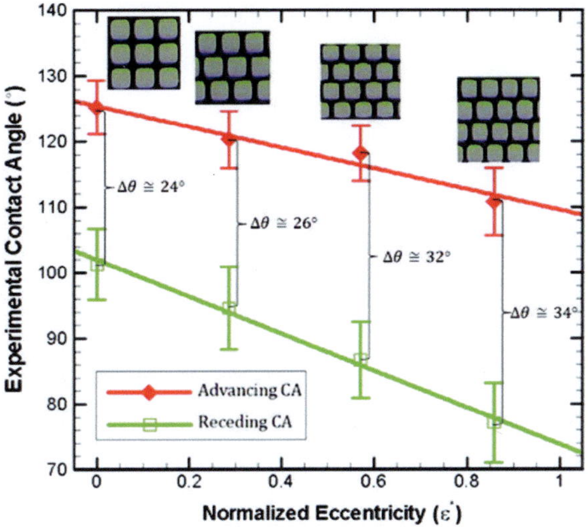

Figure 2.6.: Influence of eccentricity on the dynamic contact angle and the contact angle hysteresis.[41]

Additionally, the geometrical shape of the structures itself influence the contact angle hysteresis as described by Öner and McCarthy.[42] They examined different shapes of pillars and came to the conclusion, that by changing the shape from square to staggered rhombus, star or indented square the contact angle hysteresis is increased. This was explained by an increased pinning to the structures and a contorted contact line.

Also the distance between the structures is important. When calculating the contact angle after the Cassie-Baxter equation it is obvious that the contact angle increases with an increase in distance. The equation also shows the dependency of the contact angle in the Cassie-Baxter state of the contact angle in equilibrium, which in turn is dependent on the material.

2.4.2. Design Parameters

For biological or medical experiments a variety of materials are of interest. In this work, Cyclic Olefin Copolymer (COC) and Polysulfon (PSU) were utilized, because of their optical and biological properties. Table 2.2 shows measured advancing and receding contact angles of COC and PSU.[43]

Table 2.2.: Advancing and receding contact angles (CA) of COC and PSU

	advancing CA	receding CA
PSU	79.5 ° ± 2.3°	56.4 ° ± 0.2°
COC	97 ° ± 4.7°	73 ° ± 1.2°

The Cassie-Baxter equation was utilized to calculate the pitch of the structures. The pitch was defined as a multiple of the diameter. When calculating the contact angle after the Cassie-Baxter equation the ratio of solid-liquid to air-liquid interface is deciding. This can be calculated by the solid surface fraction f_s (Eq. 2.7)

$$f_s = \frac{f_1}{f_2} = \frac{\pi \cdot d^2}{4 \cdot p^2} \tag{2.6}$$

with p being a multiple of the diameter, the equation can be simplified to:

$$f_s = \frac{f_1}{f_2} = \frac{\pi}{4 \cdot n^2} \tag{2.7}$$

with n being a natural number greater than 1. Figure 2.7 shows the calculated contact angles for COC and PSU as well as a schematic view of the layout. The equilibrium contact angle was $\frac{\Theta_{adv}+\Theta_{rec}}{2}$.

Also replication processes were analyzed and considered for the design to allow a mass fabrication. This lead to the following proposed design.[44]

- Diameter of the structures: 10 µm to 35 µm
- Pitch of 4 · Ø(Diameter)
- Height leading to an aspect ratio of at least 2
- Checkerboard alignment

Figure 2.8 shows SEM micrographs of the fabricated microstructures. Contact angle measurements showed a superhydrophobic behavior.

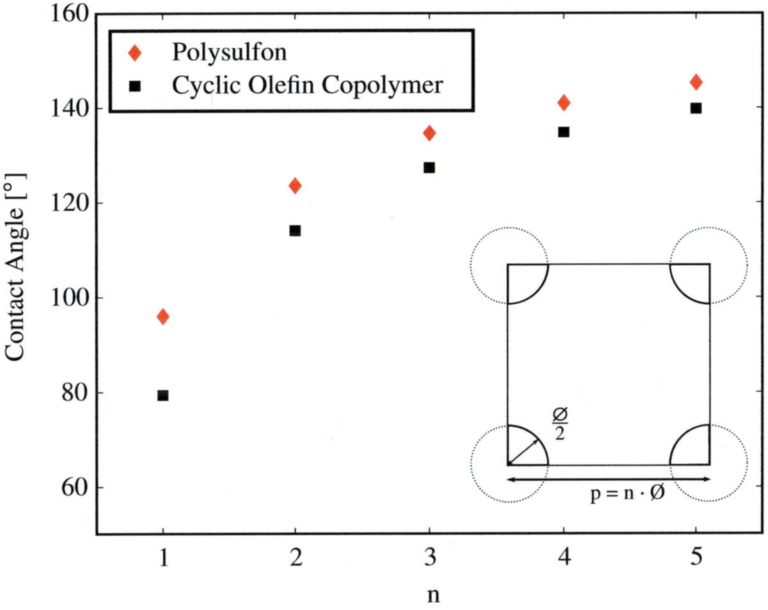

Figure 2.7.: Calculations of the contact angle after the Cassie-Baxter equation for PSU and COC. The mean value of receding and advancing contact angle was used as the equilibrium contact angle. Right lower corner: Schematic view of the Layout.

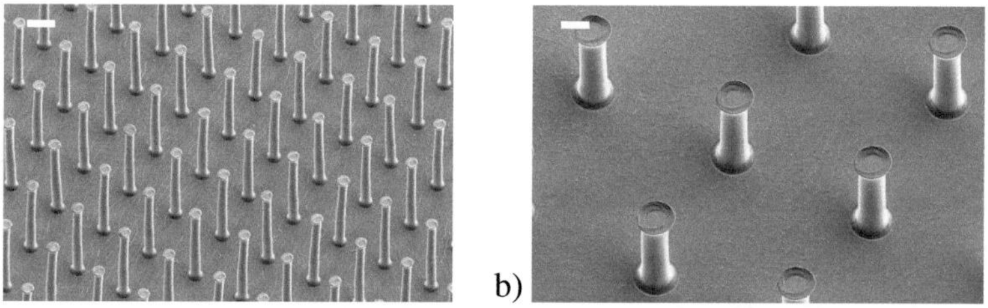
a) b)

Figure 2.8.: SEM micrographs of a) pillars with a diameter of 10 μm and a pitch of 40 μm and b) pillars with a diameter of 35 μm and a pitch of 140 μm. The height of the pillars is approx. 85 μm, which leads to aspect ratios of 8.5 and 2.4, respectively. (Scale bar: 20 μm.)

3. Fabrication Processes for Structured Microfluidic Devices

Innovation is an invention that established itself in the market.[45] To establish a product in the market in addition to demand, fabrication methods and costs are the main factors for a successful product. The demand for microfluidic systems is very high, because of their advantages against standard devices, like small analyte volumes, short detection times and easy handling. Microfluidic systems find an application in the search for new active pharmaceutical ingredients. But also in the field of medical diagnosis, *in vitro* devices or in the area of Point-of-Care (POC) diagnosis. Lab-on-a-Chip (LOC) systems reproduce the procedures in a laboratory necessary e.g. for the analysis of blood samples, on one single chip. This chip can be used directly at the patient, in rural areas or areas of conflict. These so called Point-of-Care diagnostics decrease the time of diagnosis and enable a fast and balanced treatment. However, the design of microfluidic systems does not allow mass fabrication.

Commonly in laboratory usage, LOC systems are fabricated by Polydimethylsiloxan (PDMS) molding. PDMS is a silicone based polymer, which is processed in a liquid state by mixing two viscose liquids. When the curing agent and silicone base is mixed the polymer chains of the silicone start cross-linking. Depending on the ambient temperature the polymer is still liquid for several hours, allowing an easy replication of a mold insert by pouring the mixture over the mold. When the mixture is completely cured a rubber like material is gained. This process can be accelerated by increasing the temperature. After demolding, the finished parts can be bonded to another PDMS part or to other materials like glass, by oxidizing the surface with an oxygen plasma treatment[46,47] or by using uncured PDMS as an intermediate layer.[47] PDMS devices are mainly used for short-term experiments, because it is not long-term stable. It is also often noted, that the material is insufficiently biocompatible,[48] because of its polar and hydrophobic characteristics.[49]

For mass fabrication and long-term experiments thermoplastic polymers are an interesting alternative. These materials are well characterized and a multitude of mass fabrication techniques are available, like injection molding, hot embossing and (micro-)thermoforming. Recently, these materials and fabrication techniques are gaining more and more interest.[50] Also commercialized replication machines are available for products with features in the micro-scale.[51] However, the fabrication of three-dimensional micro- and nanostructures is still highly difficult and not ready for mass fabrication. Farshchian *et al.*[52] introduced a molding technique, using a PDMS stamp to fabricate three-dimensional micro- and nanostructures. He utilized a thin PDMS stamp with nanostructures placed between a microstructured brass mold and a PMMA substrate. Afterwards a standard hot embossing process was conducted. Due to the high flexibility of the PDMS it was possible to demold even undercuts. This method is capable of replication in low-temperature polymers, because PDMS has no long-term stability at high temperatures. Therefore, only a small number of polymers are available for this method. Another method was proposed by Lim *et al.*, who combined nanoimprint lithography and focused laser beam lithography to fabricate nanopatterned microchannel molds.[53] The fabricated mold inserts can be used to replicate microchannels by UV nano imprint lithography with structures on the bottom of the channel. However, these methods still lack mass fabrication capabilities.

In this work different fabrication techniques, capable of mass fabrication, were examined and a new three-step process for the fabrication of microfluidic devices is introduced.[43] This three-step process combines hot embossing, microthermoforming and bonding to achieve three-dimensional, fully

1. Step: Hot Embossing

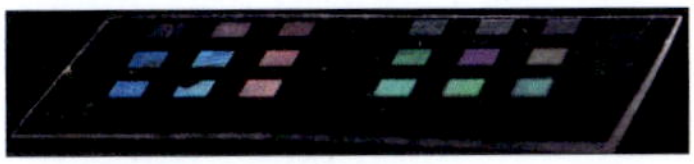

Structuring of a thin polymer foil with micro- and nanostructures.

2. Step: Microthermoforming

Drawing of the pre-structured foil into a three-dimensional shape.

3. Step: Bonding

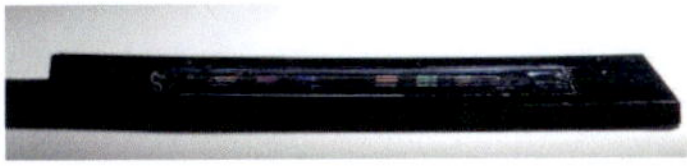

Bonding of the drawed foil onto a base plate with fluidic connectors.

Figure 3.1.: Overview of the three-step fabrication process. In the first step a thin foil is structured by hot embossing. This pre-structured foil is then brought into a three dimensional shape by microthermoforming. In the last step the thermoformed foil is bonded to a base plate with holes as fluidic connectors.[43]

structured thermoplastic polymeric parts. A schematic view of the fabrication process is shown in Figure 3.1. Additionally, injection molding is discussed as a mean of mass fabrication.

3.1. Basic Principles

Microfabrication describes the fabrication of structures where at least one dimension is in the micro-meter scale that is relevant for the function of the system. These fabrication processes can be divided into two main approaches, the top-down or bottom-up technique. The top-down approach starts with a bulk material and removes or forms material until the desired part is achieved. In the bottom-up approach the part is manufactured by arranging particles and atoms.

Depending on the used material and feature sizes the fabrication method is chosen. Many materials can be used for the fabrication of microfluidic devices. Materials are normally divided into metals and non-metal materials. Commonly silicon is used for the fabrication of micro-electro-mechanical systems (MEMS) like sensors or actuators. Recently polymers gained more and more attention because of their inexpensiveness and mass fabrication capabilities. Additionally, the wide variety of properties as well as their clearance for medical applications are of high interest.[8] Polymers can be formed by microreplication processes like hot embossing, microthermoforming and injection molding.

3.1.1. Materials

Polymeric materials can be classified into thermoplastic polymers, elastomers and thermosets.[54,55] The different classes of polymers are distinguished from each other by the network and density of polymer-chains and their thermal properties.

Thermoplastic polymers are linear or branched polymers, with no cross linking between the polymer chains. Two groups of thermoplastic polymers are known, amorphous and semi-crystalline thermoplasts. While amorphous thermoplasts have no regular arrangement of polymer chains, semi-crystalline thermoplasts have crystalline parts, with regularly arranged chains and amorphous parts with irregularly arranged chains. Both groups of thermoplastic polymers can be formed by applying heat. With an increase in temperature these materials will soften and eventual melt, enabling the processing of these polymers by various replication techniques. Thermoplastic polymers can be reheated multiple times without loosing their properties.[55,54]

Elastomers are cross-linked rubbery polymers. The network is of low cross linking density. Because of this an elastomer can be stretched up to 3-10 times of their original dimensions and, after releasing the applied stress, can spring back to its former dimensions. During stretching the polymer chains extend but are prevented from flowing by the cross-linking. They are processed in a rubbery state, where viscous flow is possible, and then vulcanized to achieve their final form.[55,56]

Thermosets have a high degree of cross-linking, which inhibits polymer chain motion, leading to a high rigidity of the material.[55,56,57] These materials will cure irreversible during heating and will be destroyed by reheating. These polymers can be formed by reactive injection molding.

In this work four thermoplastic polymers, Polycarbonate (PC), Polymethylmethacrylate (PMMA), Cyclic Olefin Copolymer (COC) and Polysulfone (PSU), were chosen, all meeting several requirements:

- Biocompatible
- Amorphous
- Good optical properties, like transparent, little or no autofluorescence
- Medical grade

PMMA is a very common polymer for prototype fabrication. This material has good optical properties and is very inexpensive. PC is a medical grade polymer with a high biocompatibility. It is often used for biological applications, especially tissue engineering. The best optical properties and no autofluorescence has COC. This polymer is therefore the best candidate for biological experiments with fluorescent biomolecules. PSU was chosen for its high chemical and temperature stability. It is autofluorescent at 248 nm but shows no autofluorescence for other wavelengths. Due to its properties this material is often used in industrial applications. Table 3.1 compares different properties of these polymers with each other.

3.1.2. Mold fabrication

Mold inserts define the quality of the fabricated part in replication processes like hot embossing, injection molding and microthermoforming. A

Table 3.1.: Properties of the utilized polymers.[57]

	PMMA	PC	COC	PSU
Density $[g/cm^3]$	1.12-1.17	1.2	1.02	1.1-1.3
Tensile strength $[N/mm^2]$	20-54	>65	66	70[58]
Elongation of break [%]	5-20	110	3-10	4-6
Young's modulus [kPa]	0.6-2.4	2.3	2.6-3.2	2.1-2.6
Service temperature				
short term [°C]	76 - 102	-115 to +150	up to 170	-50 to +180
long term [°C]	68 - 94	-115 to -130	up to 170	-50 to +150
Glass transition temp. [°C]	105[59]	150	80-180[60]	180-190
Water absorption (24h) [%]	2.1	0.15-0.3	< 0.01	0.8
Refractive index n_D^{20}	1.492	1.56-1.65	1.5	1.63-1.72[61]

mold insert contains the negative of the desired structures, which is then copied into the desired material. To avoid defects or irregularities, the mold insert as well as the fabrication is highly quality controlled. Fabrication of mold inserts is done by electrical discharge machining (EDM), laserablation, etching, mechanical micro machining or lithographic processes. The large number of fabrication processes enables the processing of different mold materials. Typically, steel, nickel, brass or aluminum are utilized for mold inserts. When using PDMS, also silicon mold inserts are employed. In this work, mechanical micro machining and the LIGA-process were utilized and will be explained in more detail.

Mechanical Micro Machining

Mechanical micro machining is used to ablate material from the bulk. Common methods are milling and drilling, which are well known from standard metal processing. They enable a fast and inexpensive fabrication of brass, aluminum or steel molds. The fabricated feature sizes are limited by the used tools. Commercially available tools are less than 22 µm.[62] Therefore, this method is commonly utilized to fabricate mold inserts for microthermoforming or hot embossing of large feature sizes like Lab-on-a-Chip systems.

Micro electrical discharge grinding (μEDM) is often used to fabricate mold inserts out of hard metals like steel or nickel. The bulk material is immersed in a dielectric medium and a high voltage is applied at the μEDM-tool, leading to a spark which in turn ablates the bulk material at the place of impact. This method leads to a rough surface[63] and is only used for large feature sizes or for post-processing of LIGA-molds.

LIGA

The LIGA (German acronym for Lithographie, Galvanik, Abformung) process describes a fabrication method consisting of lithography, electroplating and replication. In the first process step lithography is used to transfer a pattern from a mask onto a resist layer. Depending on the structure dimensions X-ray,[64] electron beam, UV-light or direct laser writing[65,66] are utilized for the lithography step. During exposure the polymer chains of a positive resist are split, leading to a reduced molecular weight. After exposure the resist is developed and exposed areas are dissolved. The substrate is then prepared for electroplating by depositing a gold electroplating starting layer by physical vapor deposition. Afterwards the substrate is placed in a nickel-electrolyte and a current is applied, leading to a growth of nickel on the starting layer. The desired thickness of the mold is depending on the utilized replication technique. Mold inserts as thin as 300 μm or 500 μm, known as Shim-Molds or Shims,[64] can be utilized for hot embossing. In general, mold inserts with a thickness of several millimeters are used.

3.2. Hot Embossing

Hot embossing, often also referred to as thermal nano imprint, is used for a precise replication of micro- or nanostructures in thermoplastic polymers.[67] This method is characterized by low residual stress in the embossed part, high flexibility, due to an easy exchange of mold inserts and material, short flow paths and an automated, precise, isothermal demolding. Because of the precise motion, force and temperature control and a high stiffness of the embossing machine structures with features of less than 100 nm can be replicated with high accuracy.

The hot embossing machine consists of a mold insert and a roughened metal plate, called substrate plate. The substrate plate is roughened by e.g. sandblasting and allows an automatic demolding due to high friction forces and therefore adhesion of the embossed part during opening of the machine. Mold insert and substrate plate are connected to heating plates, which in turn are connected to cooling blocks. The heating of the system can be done by e.g. electrical heating. In order to prevent defects and an incomplete filling of the mold cavities, due to entrapped air, the mold insert and substrate plate are surrounded by a vacuum chamber. A schematic view of the hot embossing machine is shown in Figure 3.2.

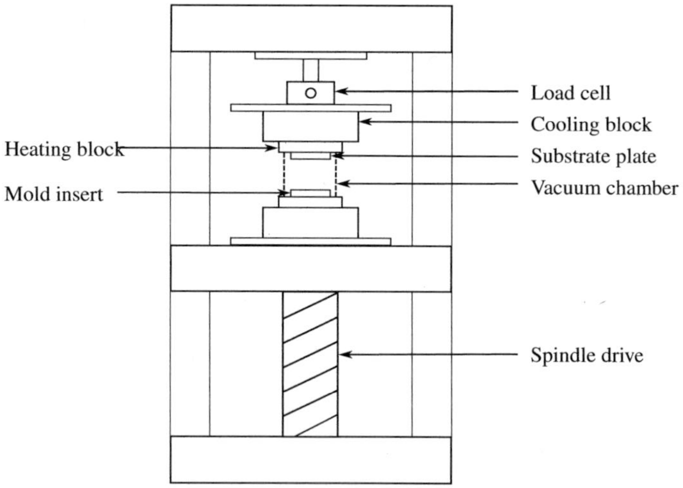

Figure 3.2.: Hot embossing setup consisting of a substrate plate and a mold insert connected to heating plates, and cooling blocks. Mounted in a stiff embossing machine with precise motion, force and temperature control. (modified after Worgull[68])

The hot embossing process can be divided into four steps:[68]

- placement of the polymer sheet and heating to the molding temperature
- establishing the molding force and pressing of the polymer into the cavities at a constant temperature
- force controlled cooling to the demolding temperature
- demolding of the finished part by opening the tool

In the first step the polymer foil is placed between a mold insert and a substrate plate. The system is closed until a touch force between 10-200 N is reached, to enable an uniform heating of the polymer. Afterwards, the mold insert is evacuated to avoid air trapping in the micro- and nanocavities. When reaching the molding temperature, the mold insert is isothermally pressed into the softened polymer foil with a high molding force. The molding force is kept constant during cooling to prevent deformations due to shrinking. Demolding occurs while opening the system. A schematic view of the hot embossing process is shown in Figure 3.3.

Hot embossing can be utilized for all thermoplastic polymers, bulk metallic glasses[69,70] and even wood.[71] Molding temperature as well as molding force are dependent on structure dimensions, material properties and structured area.

3.2.1. Experimental

Hot embossing was utilized in this work to imprint micro- and nanostructures into 50 μm to 240 μm thin thermoplastic polymer foils. PMMA and COC (TOPAS 6013 with 20% Elastomer TP140) with a thickness of 50 μm was purchased from Goodfellow. COC was additionally purchased from TOPAS with a thickness of 150 μm. PC was purchased from it4ip also with a thickness of 50 μm. PSU was available at the IMT in a thickness

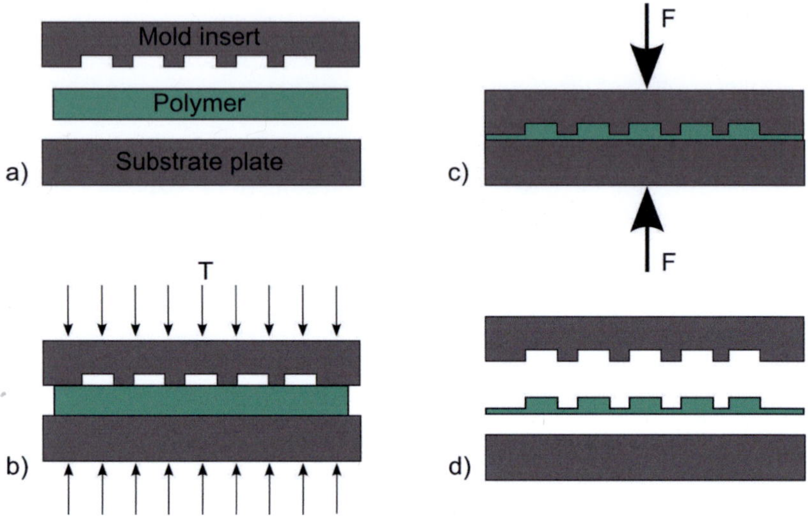

Figure 3.3.: Hot embossing process. a) A thermoplastic material is placed between a mold insert and a rough substrate plate. b) Closing of the system and heating to the molding temperature. c) Applying the molding force at a constant temperature. d) After cooling the structured polymer is demolded.

of 50 µm, 150 µm and 240 µm. Before the hot embossing process the materials were dried in a vacuum oven. This is important for hygroscopic materials, which absorb water during idle-periods. The absorbed water is then exerted during molding and evaporates, which leads to defects in the molded part. Therefore drying is recommended for polymers, especially for PSU.[57] Drying parameters are summarized in Table 3.2.

Table 3.2.: Used parameters for drying polymers in a vacuum oven.

	T [°C]	t [h]
PMMA	65	3-4
COC	80	3-4
PC	100	3-4
PSU	140	3-4

The precision of the molded parts is highly dependent on the molding temperature. The molding temperature is above the glass transition temperature of the used polymer. Figure 3.4 shows the molding windows for amorphous and semi-crystalline polymers. Amorphous polymers have a wide molding window, where the transition between the flow range and the melting state, at moderate shear modulus, occurs. For amorphous polymers these transition takes place in a wide temperature range and not at a precise temperature. Therefore, a large molding window is available. In semi-crystalline polymers crystalline and amorphous regions exists, both influencing the thermal properties of the polymer. In the glass transition range of a semi-crystalline polymer only the amorphous parts of the polymer are influenced, leading to a moderate decrease in shear modulus. By further increasing the temperature the melting range is reached. In this range the crystalline regions of the polymer melt and the polymer is changing from solid state to the melted state in a very small temperature gap of around 2 K - 3 K. This leads to a very narrow molding window.[68]

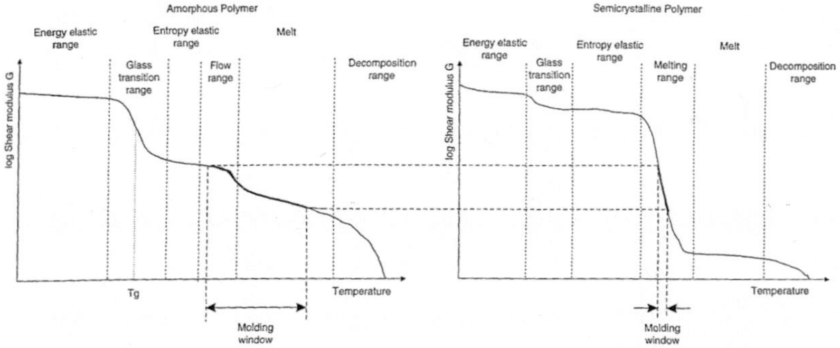

Figure 3.4.: Molding windows for amorphous and semicrystalline polymers.[68]

To characterize the thermal properties of the utilized polymers differential scanning calorimetry (DSC) was used. A sample and a reference sample are constantly heated and temperature differences are measured. These differences occur when chemical or physical changes happen, due to exothermic or endothermic reactions. The results are represented in a curve showing the heat flux over the temperature.[72] For hot embossing and microthermoforming the glass transition temperature is of great importance and was identified by these measurements. The results of these measurements can be found in Table 3.3.

The measurements also gave information about the chain formation, which was assumed to be amorphous for all polymers. This was true for PSU, PC and PMMA. But the selected type of COC was in contrast a semi-crystalline polymer. COC is a very brittle material and cannot be processed in thin foils. Therefore, elastomeric compounds are added to reduce the stiffness of the material and enable the fabrication of foils with a thickness of 50 μm. In turn these additives change the polymer formation into a semi-crystalline formation. The melting point of the elastomeric additives is very close to the glass transition temperature of the amorphous parts. This leads to a destruction of the elastomeric parts when heated to the molding temperature. The COC foils discolor and loose their elasticity. A processing of the foil by hot embossing in combination with microthermoforming is not possible. The COC foils were therefore only used for hot embossing.

Another parameter influencing the molding process is the molding force. The molding force is dependent on the aspect ratios of the cavities, the molding temperature and the structured area. Therefore depending on the different mold inserts, utilized in this work, molding forces from 40 kN to 120 kN were used.

In this work structures with features as small as 100 nm were replicated by hot embossing. Afterwards the embossed foils were examined by scanning electron microscopy as well as atomic force microscopy. Figure 3.5 shows SEM micrographs of hot embossed micro- and nanostructures.

Table 3.3.: List of hot embossing parameters with T_g being the glass transition temperature.

Material	T_g	Molding Temperature	Molding Force
PMMA	113 °C	130 °C	40 kN - 120 kN
PC	149 °C	200 °C	40 kN - 120 kN
COC	137 °C	200 °C	40 kN - 120 kN
PSU	187 °C	250 °C	40 kN - 120 kN

3.2.2. Modification A: Double sided hot embossing

For some medical applications it is very beneficial to have different micro- and nanostructures on the two sides of a polymer foil. In Chapter 4 tubes are introduced with microstructures on the inside and nanostructures on the outside, each adapted to the desired surface-surrounding interaction. To fabricate such surfaces double sided hot embossing is proposed.

This fabrication procedure is similar to a standard hot embossing process. To achieve structures on both sides of the foil, instead of a substrate plate a second mold insert was mounted into the machine. Afterwards the normal hot embossing procedure as described before was used, but with a semi-automated demolding. Typically, the molded polymer foil sticks to the substrate plate due to high friction and can then be removed. When us-

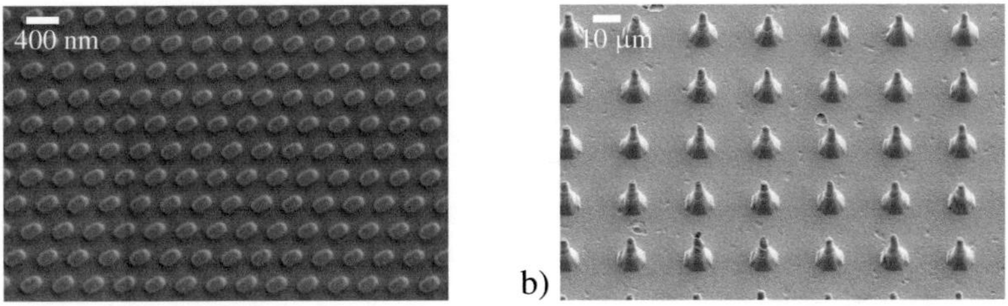

a) b)

Figure 3.5.: SEM micrograph of a hot embossed polymer foil with a) nanostructures with a cross section of 100 nm x 200 nm and a height of approx. 500 nm and b) conical microstructures with a base diameter of 10 µm and a height of approx. 25 µm.

ing two mold inserts the polymer foil will be automatically demolded from the mold with the least friction and can then be peeled off manually from the second mold insert. A SEM micrograph of a fabricated foil is shown in Figure 3.6.

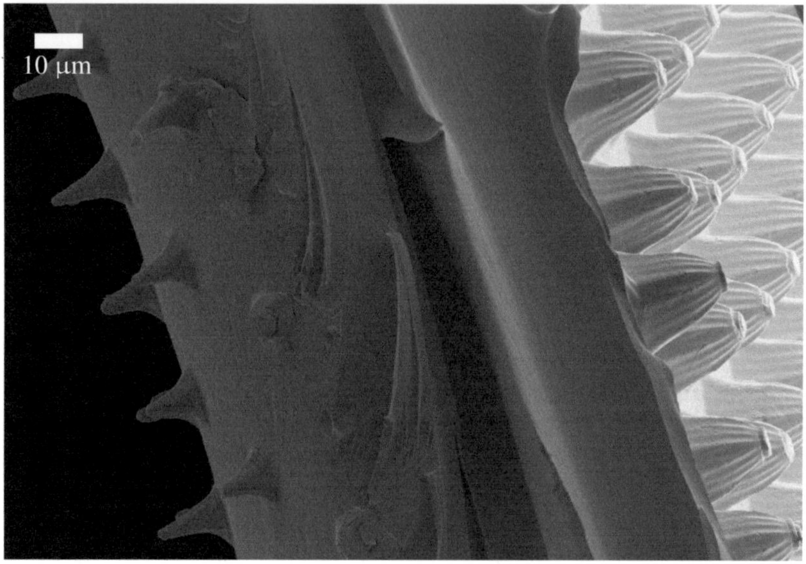

Figure 3.6.: SEM micrograph of a double sided hot embossed foil with different microstructures on the two sides.

3.2.3. Modification B: Hot Pulling

Hot pulling is a method which allows an elongation of micro- or nanostructures during the demolding step of the hot embossing process. In general, low demolding temperatures are chosen to avoid shrinkage or a deformation of the imprinted structures during demolding. Hot pulling in contrast uses high demolding temperatures to elongate the imprinted structures. At elevated demolding temperatures the material is still soft. Friction in the mold cavities sidewalls lead to adhesion inside the cavities, which combined with the soft material, leads to a deformation of the structures. Depending on the demolding temperature the length of the structures can be varied. A schematic view of the hot pulling demolding step can be found in Figure 3.7.

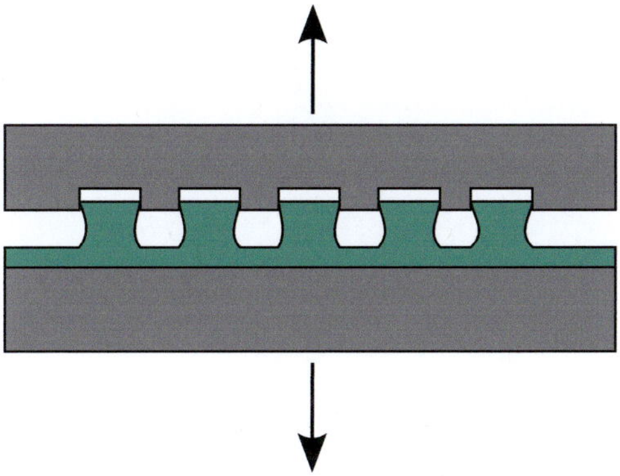

Figure 3.7.: Schematic view of the hot pulling demolding step. The still soft material is demolded at high temperatures which leads to an elongation of the structures.

This method allows the fabrication of structures higher than defined by the depth of the cavities. Aspect ratios of up to nine were achieved in this work, while the mold insert would only allow an aspect ratio of 3.5 when used with normal hot embossing parameters. Figure 3.8 shows a SEM micrograph of hot pulled micropillars. Because of the elongation during demolding the bodies of the structures are narrowed while the top of the structures have the diameter specified by the mold cavity.

Figure 3.9 compares SEM micrographs of foils fabricated with the same mold insert. Figure 3.9 a) shows incomplete structures, b) well formed structures and c) hot pulled structures.

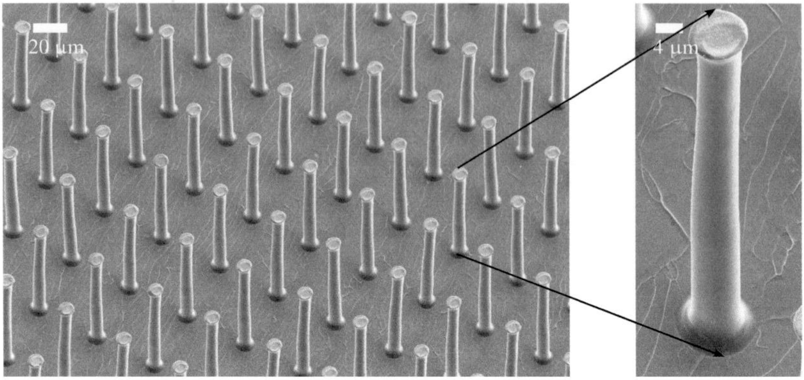

Figure 3.8.: SEM micrograph of hot pulled micro pillars with a top diameter of 9 µm and a height of 85 µm.

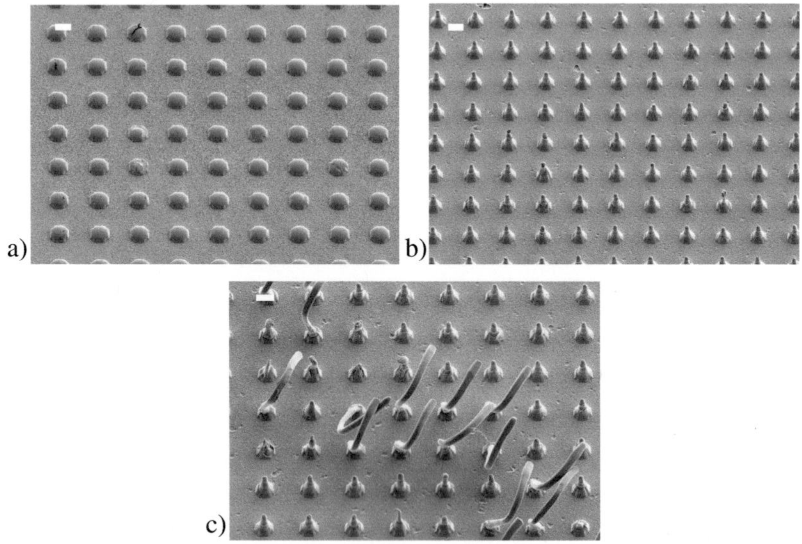

Figure 3.9.: SEM micrographs comparing the results of different molding parameters with the same mold insert and material. a) shows incomplete structures, b) fully formed structures and c) hot pulled structures. Scale bar: 10 µm.

3.2.4. Mold Insert Fabrication

In this work mold inserts fabricated by electron beam lithography and direct laser writing were utilized. Electron beam lithography was utilized for structures with diameters of 1 μm at maximum. Due to the long fabrication times of electron beam lithography, the design proposed in Chapter 2 was produced by direct laser writing. The resolution of the direct laser writing process is limited by diffraction laws and therefore much lower than for electron beam lithography. While electron beam lithography can be used to write structures with only a few nanometers in dimension, direct laser writing is used for micrometer structures. But due to the fast processing time of direct laser writers, it is a promising method for rapid fabrication and will be discussed in more detail in this section.

In the first step an anti-reflective layer, consisting of a resist with Titanium particles, is spin-coated onto a silicon wafer. This is important to avoid reflection of the laser light and therefore cross-linking of the polymer chains at undesired areas. In this work, first experiments were conducted without an anti-reflective layer, leading to a stationary wave and sandwich-like structures. Figure 3.10 shows SEM micrographs of a) micropillar without an anti-reflective layer and b) enlargement of the lower part and a micropillar c) with an anti-reflective layer and d) an enlargement of the surface.

On top of the anti-reflective layer a photosensitive resist is spin-coated. The thickness of the resist defines the height of the structures and was in this work 35 μm. The utilized resist was a negative resist named MRX-50/5100 from microresist technology. The used direct laser writer DWL66fs from Heidelberg Instruments with a Nd-YAG laser at a wavelength of 355 nm had a lateral resolution of 2.5 μm or 1 μm depending on the utilized numerical aperture. The resist is structured by scanning the laser beam over the resist. The resist is then cross-linked at the exposed areas and the structures are developed by dissolving unexposed areas. Afterwards an electro-

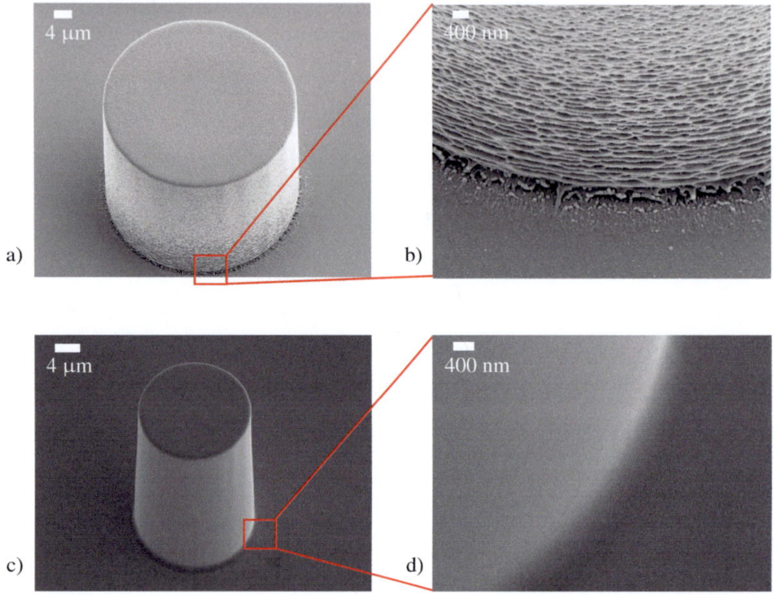

Figure 3.10.: SEM micrographs after direct laser writing a) without an anti-reflective layer of micropillars with a diameter of 22 μm and a height of 20 μm and b) an enlargement of the lower part c) with an anti-reflective layer of a micropillar with a diameter of 20 μm and a height of 20 μm d) showing an enlargement of the smooth surface.

plating starting layer, consisting of 5 nm chromium and 35 nm gold, was evaporated onto the surface. The silicon wafer was then placed into an electroplating nickel bath and nickel grew on the starting layer until a thickness of 500 μm was reached. After electroplating the silicon was removed by etching, leaving the mold insert with a thin gold and chromium layer.

3.3. Microthermoforming

In this work microthermoforming was utilized to form three-dimensional shapes, like microchannels, with micro- and nanostructured on its surfaces. Additionally, a new method named thermoformbonding was introduced, which allows thermoforming and bonding to a base plate in one process step. At the end twin-sheet-forming is discussed and utilized to form tubes with different micro- and nanostructures on the inside and outside.

Thermoforming, also known as blow molding, is a well established fabrication method in the macroscopic world, where it is used e.g. for the fabrication of car bumpers or yogurt-cups. This process utilizes pressurized gas to press a softened thermoplastic polymer foil into a mold insert. Forming of microstructures by microthermoforming is mainly used for fabricating tissue engineering scaffolds or microfluidic devices.[73,74] The microthermoforming setup is similar to the hot embossing setup and consists of a mold insert and a counter plate, both connected to heating plates and cooling blocks. These parts are implemented into a machine with precise motion control. Additionally, gas control units are installed to control gas flow and pressure. The gas is introduced into the system through gas connections and brought to the desired position through drilled holes in the mold insert.

At the beginning of the process a thermoplastic polymer foil is positioned between a mold insert and a counter plate and heated to the forming temperature while a clamping force is applied. At the forming temperature, which is around the glass transition temperature of the material, the polymer foil is pressed into the cavities by compressed gas. The gas pressure is kept constant during cooling to avoid shrinkage or spring back. After reaching the demolding temperature the system is depressurized and opened. The formed polymer is then demolded. A schematic view of the microthermoforming process is shown in Figure 3.11.

3.3.1. Experimental

Microthermoforming was used to bring 50 μm thin amorphous thermoplastic foils into a three-dimensional shape. First the foils were imprinted with micro- and nanostructures by hot embossing. Afterwards the foils were

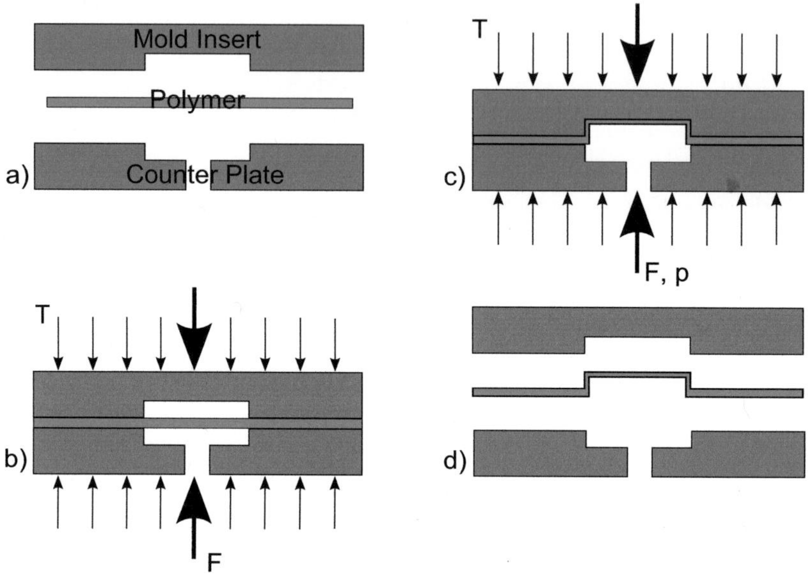

Figure 3.11.: Schematic view of the microthermoforming process. a) A thermoplastic polymer is placed between a mold insert and a counter plate. b) Closing of the system and heating to the forming temperature. c) The foil is pressed into the cavities by compressed gas. d) After cooling the formed polymer is demolded.

formed by microthermoforming by pressing the foils into the cavities by compressed nitrogen. The gas pressure was chosen after considering the size of the cavities. An increase in cavity size leads to lower gas pressure. In general, pressure between 10 and 15 bar were utilized. Figure 3.12 shows a microstructured zig-zag channel with a width of 800 μm and a height of 500 μm.

The main parameter for microthermoforming, like for hot embossing, is the forming temperature. For macroscopic thermoforming high forming temperatures, over the materials glass transition temperature, are used. This is necessary to decrease the forming pressure and to avoid spring back. For example for Polycarbonate with a glass transition temperature of 147°C

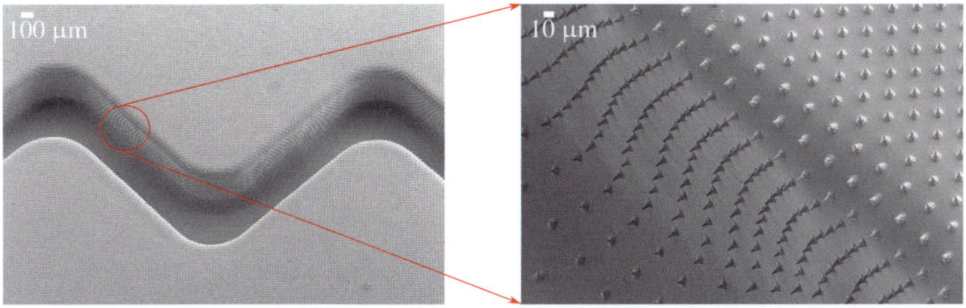

Figure 3.12.: SEM micrograph of a zig-zag channel with microstructured surfaces. The channel has a cross section of 800 μm x 500 μm, while the micropillars have a base diameter of 10 μm and a height of approx. 25 μm.

the proposed forming temperature is between 180 - 230°C.[75] In this work forming temperatures around the glass transition temperature were used to avoid destruction of the embossed structures in the foil. Therefore higher gas pressures and slightly longer cycle times were necessary to achieve a fully formed part and to avoid spring back. Forming parameters can be found in Table 3.4.

Table 3.4.: List of microthermoforming parameters.

Material	Forming Temperature	Gas Pressure
PMMA	105°C	10 - 15 bar
PC	152°C	10 - 15 bar
PSU	200°C	10 - 15 bar

3.3.2. Modification A: Thermoformbonding

In this work a new method name Thermoformbonding was introduced. This method combines microthermoforming and bonding in one process step and, therefore, enables a fast fabrication of microfluidic systems. For these experiments two mold inserts were constructed. One mold insert consisted of a workholder and gas inlets, while the other mold insert contained a cavity to from the channel as well as a broad raised section, called ridge, which completely encloses the channel cavity. The ridge will later define the bonding area.

Base plates were prepared by milling and drilling of fluidic connectors. Afterwards the base plate was placed in the workholder. The drilled fluidic connectors served as gas inlets during the thermoforming process. Over the base plate a thin thermoplastic foil was placed and the system was closed until a touch force was established. The system was then heated to the forming temperature. After reaching the forming temperature a clamping force was applied to achieve a air-tight connection between the different layers. The clamping force was thereby evenly distributed over the ridge. Then a gas pressure was applied to press the foil into the mold, forming a microchannel. Due to the heat and clamping force the foil was bonded at the defined bonding area to the base plate. A three dimensional model of the mold inserts, base plate and foil is shown in Figure 3.13.

This method enabled the forming of a channel while bonding a foil onto the base plate. During fabrication a number of challenges arose. First the size of the ridge must be chosen very carefully depending on the required clamping force. The clamping force will be evenly distributed over the ridge but for small areas it will lead to a high force per area. This in turn leads to a deformation of the base plate because the ridge imprints itself into the base plate. This can be avoided by controlling the temperature. For low temperatures, the material is still hard enough to withstand the force while for higher temperatures the ridge will easily be pressed into the base plate. Therefore, a balance between clamping force and temperature must be found.

In this work the base plate material as well as the foil material were the same polymer, because similar thermal properties are advantageous for thermobonding. However, for this proposed method different materials can be beneficial. By choosing a base plate with a higher glass transition temperature than the foil, the base plate will keep its stability while the foil is

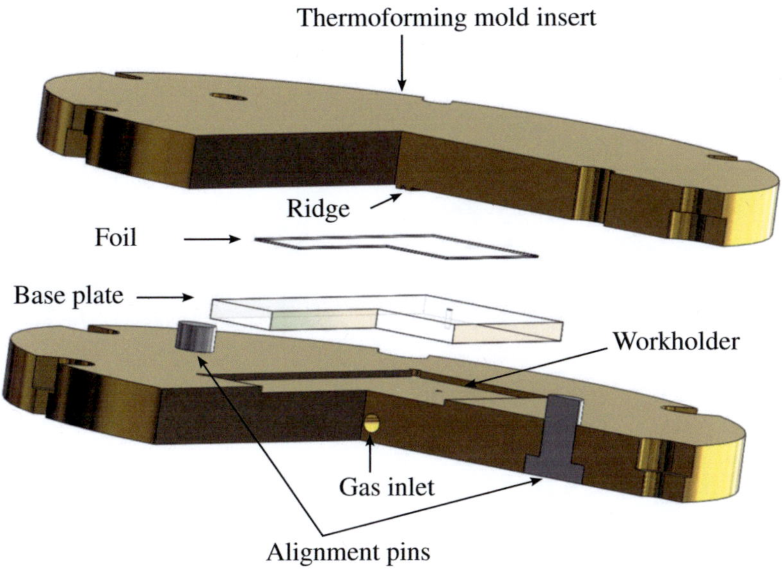

Figure 3.13.: Three dimensional model of the thermoformbonding process, consisting of a mold insert with workholder, a base plate with drilled channels, a thin foil and a microthermoforming mold insert with bonding area.

at its forming temperature. Thermobonding is meanwhile conducted at a lower temperature, but, due to the high clamping force, still possible.

3.3.3. Modification B: Twin-Sheet-Forming

To fabricate closed containers twin-sheet-forming was developed.[75] This process enables the simultaneous forming of two parts and in-process bonding. A schematic view of the process is shown in Figure 3.14. Two thermoplastic polymer foils are positioned between two mold inserts. The system is closed and heated to the forming temperature. By evacuating the mold inserts and introducing a gas pressure between the two sheets the polymer is stretched into the cavities. At the same time the two polymer sheets are bonded at the contact area, due to the heat and clamping force. The vacuum is sustained until the demolding temperature is reached. The chamber is vented and the finished part can be demolded.

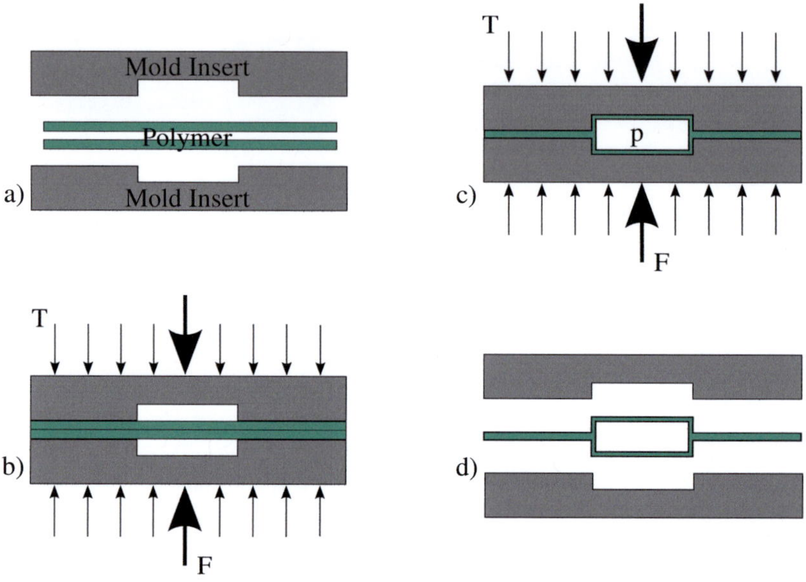

Figure 3.14.: Schematic view of the twin-sheet-forming process. a) Two polymer foils are placed between to mold inserts. b) They are clamped and heated to the forming temperature. c) The mold inserts are evacuated while a gas pressure between the two foils is build up at a constant temperature d) During cooling the gas pressure is kept constant to avoid shrinkage or spring back. After reaching the demolding temperature the system is opened and the formed part can be demolded.

The gas pressure between the two foils can be introduced in several ways. For closed chambers a material is brought between the two foils which will evaporate at the forming temperature. In this work a mold insert was constructed with an implemented gas inlet, which guides the gas between the two foils. This enabled the fabrication of micropipettes and tubes (see Chapter 4).

3.4. Bonding

Bonding is defined as the joining of two parts. A wide variety of bonding methods are available for polymer microsystems, like adhesive bonding, welding and solvent bonding.[76,77] For polymer parts with large features conventional welding techniques, like laser welding, ultrasonic welding or infrared welding, can be used.

In this work laser welding, thermobonding and adhesive bonding were used to bond a microthermoformed foil to a base plate to achieve a liquid tight channel. First prototypes were bonded by gluing, which is an easy to use and quick method. This method also allows to join two different materials. Laser welding and thermobonding were utilized because of their capability for mass production. For thermobonding as well as laser welding materials with the same thermal properties are beneficial. Therefore, these processes were used to join the same type of material (PC-PC or PSU-PSU).

3.4.1. Adhesive Bonding

This bonding method utilizes an adhesive between two parts. Typically, two component adhesives are used. They can be applied by capillary forces, laminating processes or by filling of special channels. Adhesive bonding by capillary forces is often combined with UV-light curable adhesives. After the adhesive is introduced into the capillaries, UV-light is utilized to cross-link its polymer chains, which leads to an immediate hardening of the adhesive. Lamination is used for large area bonding and leads to a thin adhesive layer between two parts. When clearly defined bonding areas are necessary, channels for adhesives can be implemented into the microfluidic chip. The adhesive is then injected into the channels and after a complete filling can be cured by UV-light or heat. However, all methods have to be processed carefully to avoid that the adhesive enters the microfluidic channel which would lead to clogging and contamination of the channel.

In this work microthermoformed channels were bonded onto a base plate with fluidic connectors. A UV-curable adhesive, Delo Photoond PB437, was laminated onto the base plate. Afterwards the microthermoformed channels were placed on the base plate and positioned under an UV-light source. After 90 seconds the adhesive was cured and a bond between channel and base plate was achieved. These parts were used in this work for fluidic experiments (see Chapter 4) and for protein adsorption experiments (see Chapter 5).

3.4.2. Thermobonding

Thermobonding uses heat and pressure to achieve a tight joining of two materials. Due to the heat an increase in molecule motion takes place. This leads to an inter-diffusion of the polymer chain. The bond strength possible to acquire with this method can be as high as the drag-strength of the material itself.

In this work thermobonding was used for preliminary tests to the thermoformbonding process. Therefore two polished plates were mounted into the hot embossing machine. The base plate and a foil was positioned in the machine and the system was closed until a touch force was reached. The system was than heated to a temperature slightly over the glass transition temperature. A bonding force was isothermally applied and kept constant for five minutes. Afterwards the system was cooled and the bonding force reduced. These experiments were conducted with COC, utilizing a bonding temperature of 140°C and a bonding force of 20 kN.

3.4.3. Laser Welding

Laser welding was used to bond the base plate to the microthermoformed channel. This method is widely used in industrial fabrication processes. A schematic view of the process is shown in Figure 3.15 For this process a transparent and a laser light absorbing polymer are needed. Therefore, a base plate material with carbon additives was utilized. The two polymer parts are clamped together and a laser beam is scanned over the desired weld seam. The laser light is absorbed by the polymer with carbon additives and the polymer is melted. The heat is then transferred to the other polymer and the two molten materials fuse together. After cooling a liquid tight bond is achieved. In this work a diode laser with a wavelength of 940 nm and a maximum power density of 0.38 mW/μm² was used.

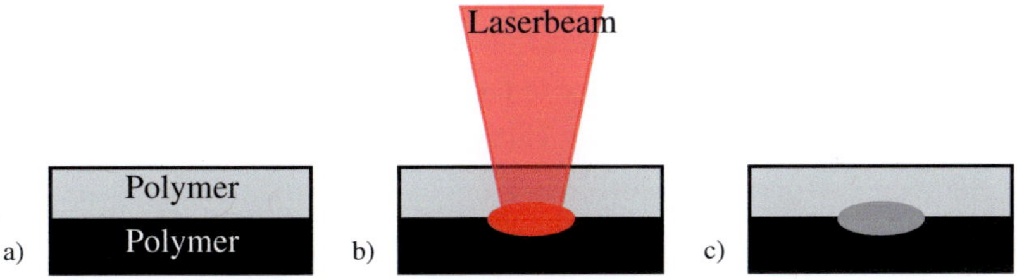

Figure 3.15.: a) A transparent and a laser light absorbing polymer are clamped together. b) Laser light is adsorbed by the lower polymer and heated to its melting temperature. c) By heat transport the transparent polymer is also heated and both polymers are welded together.

3.5. Injection Molding

Injection molding is the most common process for large batch fabrication of identical parts. It is used to fabricate automotive parts, packing, household articles, consumer electronics goods and toys. It is the main industrial fabrication process for thermoplastic, duroplastic and elastomeric parts. Its greatest advantage is the high reproducibility as well as low cycle times. Due to its high importance in industrial manufacturing it is also a well studied process.[78,79]

An injection molding machine consists of a hopper, heated screw, nozzle and a mold insert. The process can be divided into three major steps:[80]

- Injection Phase
- Plastification
- Ejection

Figure 3.16 shows a simplified view of the injection molding setup. Granular polymer is filled into a hopper and moved by gravity into the screw. The screw is moving the material to the nozzle while it gets heated. When it reaches the nozzle the polymer is in a melted state. The preset injection volume at the tip of the screw is injected by a forward push of the screw, through a nozzle into the closed mold. For traditional injection molding, mold temperatures between room temperature and 80 °C are commonly used.[80] For mold inserts with both large and very small features, this can lead to an uneven filling of the mold insert and defects. Because of the low temperature the material will cool down instantaneously when in contact with the mold insert, especially at areas with a large surface to volume ratio. This can lead to blocking of channels and an uneven filling of the mold insert. To avoid these defects, higher mold temperatures are preferred.

Additionally, the rapid cooling of the material leads to high stresses inside fabricated parts. These stresses can lead to poor post-processing results, for example when used for different bonding processes. Therefore, a combination of hot embossing and injection molding can be used, called injection compression molding. This method is also using a screw to convey and heat the polymer until it is melted. It is then injected into a mold insert, which is not completely closed. The two halves will close after the injection and can be motion and velocity-controlled. This leads to an even distribution of the pressure, small flow paths and to less stress inside the material. Injection compression molding is commonly utilized to fabricate CDs and DVDs.

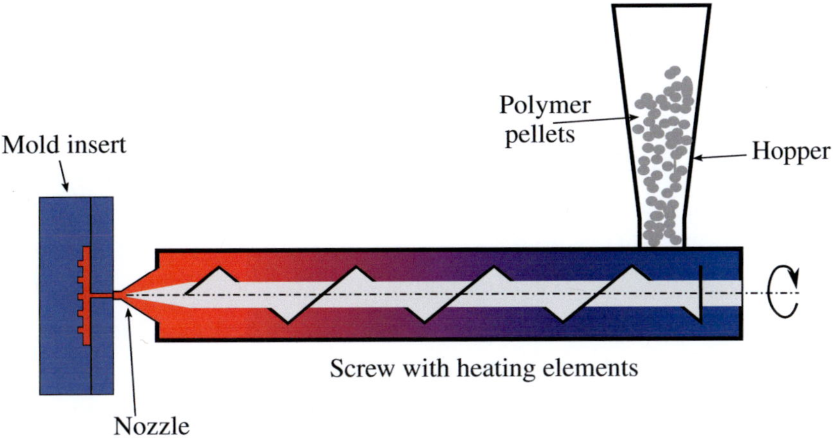

Figure 3.16.: Simplified view of the injection molding setup. Polymer pellets are fed to a screw to convey the material to the nozzle while it gets heated. A injection volume is injected by a forward motion of the screw. The material solidifies within a few seconds in the mold insert and gets ejected by pins.

Since the 1990s micro-injection molding is getting commercialized. This process is defined as an injection molding process with injection volumes of less than 1 cm^3. Add-ons as well as micro-injection molding setups are commercially available.

In this work injection molding was utilized to fabricate half-finished parts for hot embossing and fluidic base plates.

3.6. Discussion and Outlook

The fabrication of LOC systems is a vital part for the advancement of these systems. Especially for the use in POC diagnostics robust and disposable devices are necessary. This work focused not only on the design of a new system but also on a simple and cost effective method of its fabrication. Therefore, different fabrication methods were utilized and analyzed to find a suitable candidate for the proposed applications.

Hot embossing enabled a precise replication of structure features down to 100 nm. Because of the low stresses inside the material, structured foils were easily post-processed by microthermoforming and/or bonding. Process cycle times were around 5 to 10 minutes and therefore adequate for small and medium batch fabrication. This process is extremely flexible, not only because of the easy change of mold inserts, but also because of the fast change of processing material.

On the other hand, the proposed chip design is capable of being replicated by injection molding or injection compression molding. These processes are characterized by very low cycle times (below 1 minute) and no residual layer. The drawbacks compared to hot embossing are easily overcome when fabricating large batch series. This can be experienced everyday when listening to music or watching a movie from a DVD or CD. These products possess macrofeatures as well as features with only a few nanometers. Despite this wide field of application it is still not possible to fabricate fully structured three dimensional shapes, due to the demolding step.

Microthermoforming on the other hand is well suited for fabricating three-dimensional shapes. The dimensions of the fabricated channels is limited by the thickness of the polymer foil. The thickness of the foil also greatly influences handling, which makes the bonding to a rigid base plate for most applications inevitable. Because of low forming temperatures compared to the hot embossing molding temperatures this method opens unique possibilities in combination with hot embossing.

4. Properties and Applications of Structured Microfluidic Devices

The combination of hot embossing and microthermoforming enables the fabrication of structured channels enabling a passive control of fluids. In this chapter the influence of surface structures on wetting behavior as well as on dynamic fluid behavior is analyzed and further applications in medicine are introduced.

4.1. Measurement of the Wetting Behavior

Contact angle measurements are typically used to gain information about the wetting behavior of a surface. Either static contact angle measurements or dynamic contact angle measurements can be performed. Static contact angle measurements can have a large variance. This is dependent on the adhesion of the droplet on the surface. Therefore, dynamic contact angle measurements are used to get a more precise image of the wetting behavior. In this work both methods for measuring the contact angle were utilized, depending on the size of the structured area.

4.1.1. Experimental Setup

Static and dynamic contact angle measurements were conducted with a DataPhysics OC20 setup. This setup consists of a syringe connected to a controller, a light source, to achieve a high contrast between the droplet and the surface, a microscope with a camera and a computer with an analysis program. A schematic view of the setup is shown in Figure 4.1. For all experiments water was used as the testing fluid.

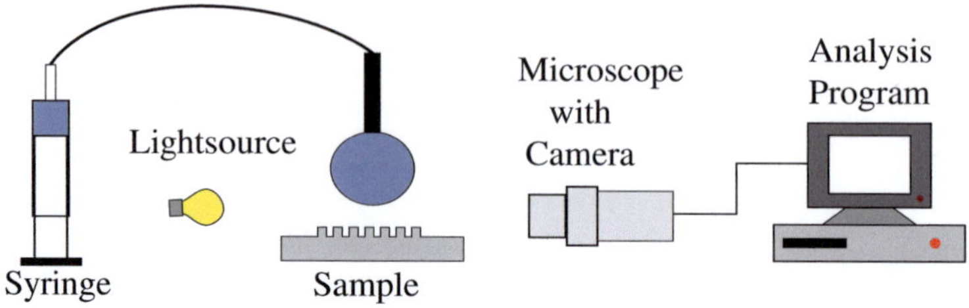

Figure 4.1.: Schematics of the contact angle measurement setup. A drop is dispensed by a syringe on the sample. An image is taken by a microscope and analyzed by a computer program.

For static contact angle measurements a water droplet of 1.5 μl was dispensed and the angle between water droplet and surface was measured. All contact angle measurements were carried out in cleanroom environment with a temperature of 24.7 °C ± 0.8 °C and a humidity of 13.6 % RH ± 1 % RH. For dynamic contact angle measurements the sessile drop needle in method was used. A droplet was dispensed on the surface with the needle still inside the droplet. The volume of the droplet was increased with a flow rate of 0.2 μl/s to a total volume of 10 μl. Contact angle measurements were performed constantly. During the increase of the volume the droplet increases its size but at the same time keeps the area of surface contact stable until the advancing contact angle is reached. This is the maximum contact angle at which the surface tension is at an equilibrium with the pinning force. A further increase in volume leads to a sudden movement of the triple line and an increase of contact area. This movement of the triple line will take place at the same contact angle each time. The receding contact angle is measured while decreasing the drop volume with a rate of 0.2 μl/s. Again the contact area will stay constant until the receding contact angle is reached, leading to a sudden movement of the triple line and a decrease of the contact area. For all samples three measurements were taken and the mean value as well as the standard deviation were calculated. The manufacturer of the measurement setup recommends a different measurement approach. When the maximum volume is reached a waiting time is implemented before decreasing the volume. During this waiting time a stable contact angle ensues. This contact angle is then taken as the advancing contact angle.

4.1.2. Results and Discussion

Dynamic contact angle measurements were utilized to analyze the dependency of the contact angle on the material by structuring polymeric surfaces with octagonal conical structures. The structured have a base diameter of 10 μm, a height of approximately 25 μm and a pitch of 25 μm. The results as well as a SEM micrograph of the microstructures are shown in Figure 4.2. The results show the advancing and receding contact angles of the unstructured material (black) and of the structured material (corresponding icons in red). For all materials an increase of around 20 ° is observed. The contact angle hysteresis is not changing significantly for all samples.

These experiments are in conflict with the Wenzel theory. The Wenzel theory states, that a hydrophilic material can not change into a hydrophobic material by changing the surface roughness. These experiments show, that for all utilized materials, a change of wetting behavior from the hydrophilic regime into the hydrophobic regime was possible.

To examine the influence of pitch and diameter on the contact angle COC foils were structured with circular pillars with a diameter of 250 nm, 500 nm and 750 nm, a height of 1 μm and a pitch of n·Ø with n=2..5. After the experiments, theoretical contact angles after the Wenzel theory were calculated and compared to the results. Because the Wenzel equation does not allow a hydrophilic material to become hydrophobic, the utilized equilibrium contact angle was taken as the advancing contact angle of COC and was 97 °. In Figure 4.3 the results for the theoretical measurements (bold lines) and experimental results (dotted lines) are shown. For a pitch of more than 3·Ø the results are in good agreement with the theoretical values. For a smaller pitch the contact angles are higher than the calculated values. A

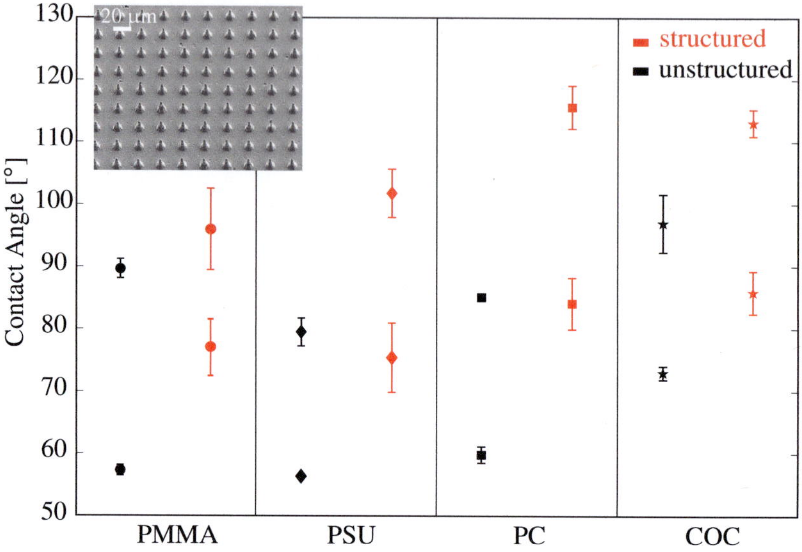

Figure 4.2.: Dynamic contact angle measurements of PMMA, PSU, PC and COC. Black icons show the advancing (upper) and receding (lower) contact angle of the unstructured polymer foil. The corresponding red icons show the advancing and receding contact angle of the structured polymer foil (SEM micrograph of the structures is shown in the upper left corner). The contact angle increases by about 20 ° for all materials. The absolute value is dependent on the unstructured materials contact angle. The contact angle hysteresis is not changing significantly.

possible explanation is, that the fluid is not in the Wenzel state but in either a metastable or stable Cassie-Baxter state. Therefore higher contact angles are possible. Experiments with the same structures and other polymers were conducted and showed similar results.

Contact angle measurements are a difficult task to perform. When measuring the dynamic contact angle of a surface the advancing contact angle is often obvious and therefore easy to measure. In contrast, the receding contact angle is highly dependent on the adhesion of the surface as well as the state of the fluid. For fluids in the Wenzel state a high contact angle

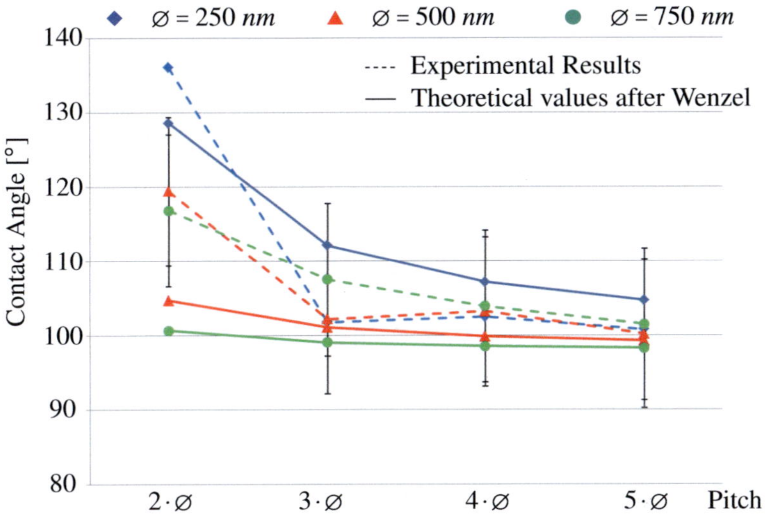

Figure 4.3.: Static contact angle measurements of COC in comparison with calculated contact angles after the Wenzel-Theory. For pitches of over 3·Ø the measured contact angles are in good agreement with the theoretical values. For a pitch of 2·Ø the contact angles are larger, this can be described by a fluid in the Cassie-Baxter state.

hysteresis is measured because of the large area of contact and therefore high adhesion between the fluid and the surface. This leads to a very low receding contact angle, which is often immeasurable.

Static measurements are taken from a sessile drop on the surface. A liquid drop will constantly evaporate, leading to a change in size and contact angle. Therefore, the time between dispension and measurement should be as short as possible. Additionally, the speed of evaporation is highly dependent on the temperature as well as the humidity. High contact angles are often measured at a high humidity. This effect is playing a minor role in the presented results, because all experiments were conducted in a cleanroom environment with temperature and humidity control.

Surfaces leading to a metastable Cassie-Baxter state can be disturbed easily. Vibrations or a draft can lead to a transition from the Cassie-Baxter state to the Wenzel state and involves a sudden decrease in contact angle.

4.2. Dynamic Fluid Behavior

The introduced combination of fabrication processes allow the production of fully structured microchannels. The structures on the surface can influence the dynamic fluid behavior by changing e.g. the friction. Different methods are available to measure the behavior of fluids inside microchannels. Often particles are introduced into a channel and used to visualize velocity vectors by tracking these particles. This method is known as particle image velocimetry or particle tracking velocimetry. Additionally, pressure loss experiments are used to evaluate friction inside a channel. In this work micro astigmatism particle tracking velocimetry (μAPTV) was utilized to gain information about the velocity profiles of water in a micro- or nanostructured channel. These measurements were conducted in cooperation[1] with the Institute of Fluid Dynamics and Aerodynamics at the Universität der Bundeswehr München.[81]

4.2.1. Theory and State of the Art

The fluid flow inside a channel can be divided into two types, laminar flow and turbulent flow. A laminar flow is characterized by a straight particle path parallel to the channel walls.[82] Mixing of fluids in the laminar flow is only possible through diffusion. For turbulent flows the flow is unsteady and a particle will move chaotically inside the channel. When analyzing the velocity profiles for these two types a clear distinction can be made. A laminar flow is characterized by a parabolic shape with a large velocity gradient at the wall, while a turbulent flow has a small velocity gradient and an almost even velocity distribution. Additionally, the mean velocity and the

[1] Data was obtained and made available from S. Schillo (IMT)

maximum velocity for turbulent flow are closer together. The low velocity at the channel walls or the zero velocity in laminar flow, respectively, is due to shear stress on the wall. A schematic view of the laminar and turbulent velocity flows are shown in Figure 4.4.

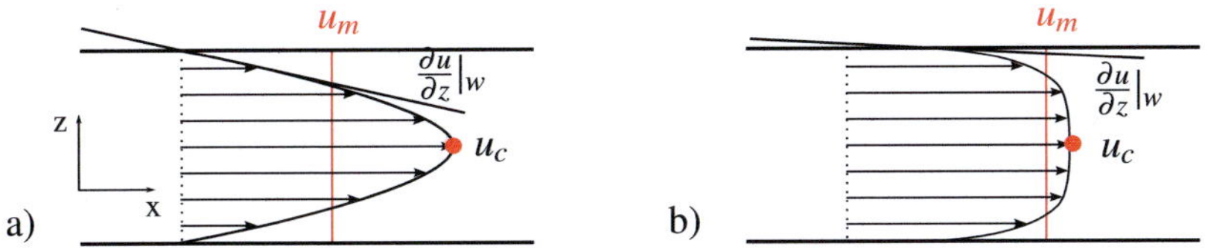

Figure 4.4.: Velocity profile in a channel with a fluid in a) laminar flow and b) turbulent flow.

By using the dimensionless Reynolds number the flow behavior can be calculated. At a Reynolds number of $Re < 2300$ the flow is defined as laminar, while higher Reynolds numbers describe a turbulent flow. The Reynolds number Re is defined as the ratio between inertial force and the viscous force and is described by the mean velocity u_m (see Figure 4.4), the density of the fluid ρ, the hydraulic diameter d_h and the dynamic viscosity η (Eq. 4.1):

$$Re = \frac{u_m \rho d_h}{\eta} \tag{4.1}$$

The hydraulic diameter for rectangular microchannels is defined as $d_h = \frac{4A}{U}$, with the cross-section area $A = H \cdot B$ and the wetted circumference $U = 2 \cdot (H + B) \cdot l$, with H being the height, B the width and l the length of the microchannel. In microfluidics the channel dimensions are very small (in this work $H < 450 \mu m$ and $B < 700 \mu m$). For water at 25 °C the dynamic viscosity is $\eta_w = 0.891 \cdot 10^{-3} \frac{kg}{m \cdot s}$ [83] and the density is $997.05 \frac{kg}{m^3}$, which would lead to a turbulent flow for a mean velocity of $u_m > 3.75 \frac{m}{s}$ which corresponds to a volume flow $\dot{V} = u_m \cdot A$ of $\dot{V} = 1.2\frac{ml}{s}$. In this work, volume flows of $\dot{V} < 3\frac{\mu l}{s}$ were used. Therefore, for all experiments a laminar flow can be assumed.

The motion of a fluid is described by the Navier-Stokes equations. These equations combine the continuity equation (Eq. 4.2) and balance of momentum (Eq. 4.4) to describe a viscous flow.

$$\frac{\mathrm{D}}{\mathrm{D}t}(\delta m_R) = \frac{\mathrm{D}\rho}{\mathrm{D}t} + \rho\frac{\partial u_i}{\partial x_i} = 0 \tag{4.2}$$

For incompressible flows:

$$\frac{\mathrm{D}\rho}{\mathrm{D}t} = 0 \tag{4.3}$$

$$\rho\frac{\mathrm{D}u_j}{\mathrm{D}t} = \rho f_j + \frac{\partial \tau_{ij}}{\partial x_i} \tag{4.4}$$

with τ being the shear stress for Newtonian fluids (Eq. 4.5) with the strain rate tensor e_{ij} (Eq. 4.6), which includes the velocity gradient.

$$\tau_{ij} = -p\delta_{ij} + 2\eta e_{ij} \tag{4.5}$$

$$e_{ij} = \frac{1}{2}\left(\frac{\partial u_i}{\partial x_j} + \frac{\partial u_j}{\partial x_i}\right) \tag{4.6}$$

leading to the Navier-Stokes equation:

$$\rho\left(\frac{\partial u_j}{\partial t} + u_i\frac{\partial u_j}{\partial x_i}\right) = -\frac{\partial p}{\partial x_j} + \eta\frac{\partial^2 u_j}{\partial x_j \partial x_i} + \rho f_j \tag{4.7}$$

For steady, fully developed flows the Navier-Stokes equation can be simplified to:

$$\rho\left(u_i\frac{\partial u_j}{\partial x_i}\right) = -\frac{\partial p}{\partial x_j} + \eta\frac{\partial^2 u_j}{\partial x_i \partial x_i} \tag{4.8}$$

with further simplification for laminar flow the Navier-Stokes equation in x-direction:

$$0 = -\frac{\partial p}{\partial x} + \eta \frac{\partial^2 u}{\partial z^2} \tag{4.9}$$

In microfluidics surface effects, like friction, highly influence the fluid behavior because of the large surface to volume ratio. To calculate friction losses two theories can be used. First the Navier-Stokes equation can be utilized to calculate the Darcy friction factor c_f (Eq. 4.10), a dimensionless factor that correlates the wall shear stress with the kinetic energy. To calculate this factor, information about the velocity gradient is necessary and can be gained from the shear stress at the wall τ_w (Eq. 4.11).

$$c_f = \frac{\tau_w}{\frac{\rho}{2} u_m^2} \tag{4.10}$$

with

$$\tau_w = \eta \left. \frac{\partial u}{\partial z} \right|_w \tag{4.11}$$

Another possibility is to use the flow filament theory to calculate, by taking the Bernoulli equation (Eq. 4.12) into account, the Fanning friction factor λ (Eq. 4.13). When using this theory, information about the pressure drop $\triangle p_v$ is required.

$$\frac{\rho}{2} u_m^2 + p + \rho g h + \triangle p_v = const. \tag{4.12}$$

with

$$\triangle p_v = \frac{\rho}{2} u_m^2 \frac{l}{d_h} \lambda \tag{4.13}$$

For a rectangular channel cross section and laminar flow the Darcy friction factor can be theoretically calculated with Eq. 4.14.

$$c_f = \varphi \cdot \frac{64}{Re} = \frac{1}{4} \lambda \tag{4.14}$$

The constant φ is dependent on the width and height of the channel and can either be calculated numerically[82] or found in literature.[84, 85]

Hetsroni *et al.*[86] reported an inconsistency between theoretical values and experimental data and gives three main influencing factors for this behavior:

- measurement errors
- discrepancy between experimental conditions and theoretical assumptions
- effects, due to the miniaturization and therefore larger surface to volume ratio

Also an effect called slip-condition is additionally playing a role in these systems. In general the velocity at the solid-liquid boundary is assumed to be zero. However, due to trapped air between structures on the surface, the fluid slips over areas of entrapped air, leading to a velocity unequal to zero. Because these areas of slip and no slip are not distinguishable from each other when analyzing the fluid behavior, a velocity at the solid-liquid boundary is measured, being the average of no slip and slip velocities. This can also be quantified by the slip length λ, which defines the deviations from the no slip condition.[87] Additionally, slip can also be achieved when a gas layer between surface and liquid is achieved. A schematic depiction of these conditions are shown in Figure 4.5.

4.2.2. Experimental Setup

The particle movement was measured by micro astigmatism particle tracking velocimetry (µAPTV). In this work polystyrene particles with a diameter of 5 µm and a fluorescence label emitting at a wavelength of 607 nm purchased from Microparticles GmbH were utilized. The fluorescence dye of the particles was excited with a Nd:YAG Litron laser with a wavelength of 532 nm in double pulse mode. The laser light excites the fluorescence particles and the emitted light passes through a microscope and is diverted

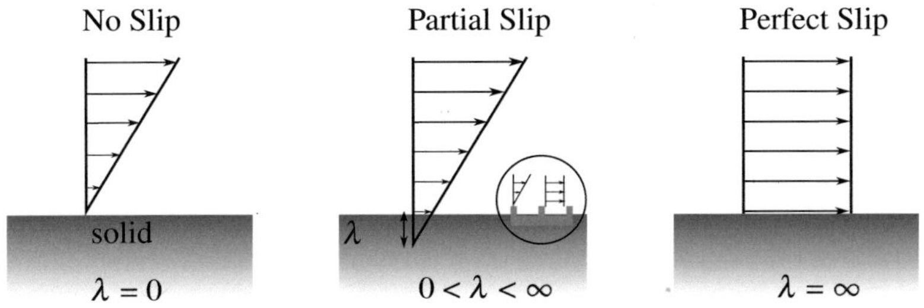

Figure 4.5.: Schematic view of the no-slip, partial-slip and slip condition and the corresponding velocities, with λ being the slip length. (modified from Tropea *et al.*[87])

at a dichroic beam splitter to a PCO.edge sCMOS camera. To get three-dimensional information about the velocity vectors a cylindrical lens is introduced into the light pass, leading to two separated focal planes. The distance of the focal planes are determined by the focal length of the utilized cylindrical lens. The detected particle images appear elliptical distorted, giving information about the z-component of the velocity (from the axis-length of the ellipse). By tracking the center location of the particle, information about the x- and y-components are gained. A schematic view of the setup is shown in Figure 4.6.[88]

Three differently structured channels were utilized as well as an unstructured channel. The channels had an outer dimension of 500 μm by 800 μm and a length of 35 mm, and were fabricated by combining hot embossing, microthermoforming and adhesive bonding. For bonding the UV-curable adhesive Delo-Photobond PB437 was utilized. To connect the channels to a syringe pump, PC tubes were glued into the channel by using the UV-curable adhesive. Table 4.1 summarizes the dimensions of the channels and structures.

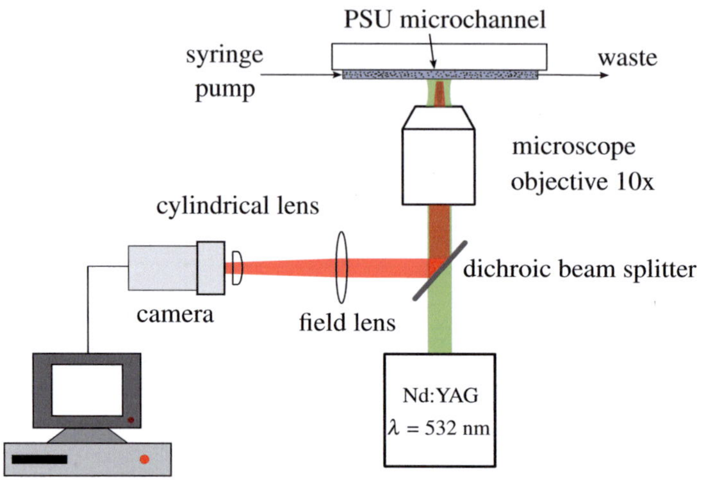

Figure 4.6.: Schematic view of the μAPTV setup. Laser beam with a wavelength of 532 nm passes through a microscope objective into the microchannels. Polystyrene particles are excited and fluorescence light is reflected and diverted by a dichroic beam splitter through a field lens and a cylindrical lens into a camera. (modified from Cierpka and Kähler[88])

Table 4.1.: Summary of utilized structures and channel dimensions with H being the Height, W being the Width of the channel, p being the pitch, d the diameter and h being the height of the structures.

structures	H × W [μm]	d_h [μm]	p [μm]	d [μm]	h [μm]
unstructured	425 × 650	514	none	none	none
circular	426 × 652	515.3	0.5	0.25	0.5
conical	495 × 690	576.5	25	10	25
ellipsoid	426 × 652	515.3	0.4	0.12 × 0.24	0.5

4.2.3. Results

Velocity profiles as well as SEM micrographs of the corresponding surface structures are shown in Figure 4.7. The data was analyzed and a curve was fitted through the data by using a polynomial fit second degree. A measurement error of 5 % was assumed and is depicted by the errorbars. Table 4.2 shows the mean velocity, Reynolds number and Darcy friction factor calculated from the µAPTV measurements.

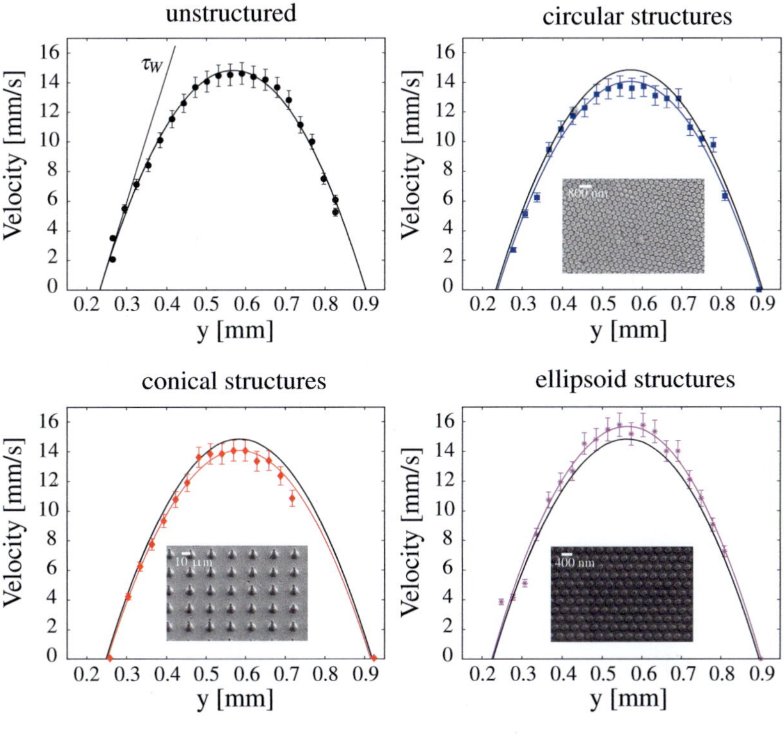

Figure 4.7.: Velocity profiles of differently structured channels, imaged by µAPTV. An error of 5 % is assumed and depicted by the errorbars. The black curve in the structured diagrams represents the fitted velocity profile of the unstructured channel.[81] Additionally, SEM micrographs show the utilized structures.

Because the velocity profiles do not sufficiently describe the friction behavior, the Darcy friction factor as well as the Reynolds numbers for the four different samples were calculated from the measured data. Table 4.2 summarizes, while Figure 4.8 shows a Nikuradse diagram of the results.

Table 4.2.: Mean velocity, Reynolds number and Darcy friction factor calculated from the results of the μAPTV measurements.

structures	$u_m = \frac{u_c}{2}$	Re	c_f
unstructured	7.3 $\frac{mm}{s}$	4.2	2.67
circular	6.9 $\frac{mm}{s}$	3.96	2.84
conical	6.7 $\frac{mm}{s}$	4.51	3.1
ellipsoid	7.9 $\frac{mm}{s}$	4.55	2.46

The theoretical values are calculated after Eq. 4.14 with $\varphi = 0.93$.[85] The Nikuradse diagram visualizes the correlation between Reynolds number and Darcy friction factor. The errorbars depict an error of 10% in the Darcy friction factor and 5% of the Reynolds number. While channels with conical structures have the lowest Reynolds number, the measured Darcy friction factor is higher than for all other samples. All results are below the theoretical value, giving the impression of a decrease in friction for all channels. Because this cannot be the case for the unstructured channels, the most likely explanation is a systematic measurement error. This could be either problems with the velocity measurements or with the measurements of the hydraulic diameter.

Also contact angle measurements of the utilized structures were conducted. Table 4.3 summarizes the results of dynamic contact angle measurements for the structures, showing the receding and advancing contact angle as well as the contact angle hysteresis. Especially the contact angle hysteresis is very important, because it characterizes the adhesion of a droplet on a surface. For the utilized structures this would lead to the conclusion of a low friction for microchannels with conical structures, because of the high contact angles and low contact angle hysteresis. This is in good agreement with the measured data. No difference between the other channels can be measured.

Two factors could influence the differences in theoretical behavior and measured data. First, the liquid is in a metastable Cassie-Baxter state and

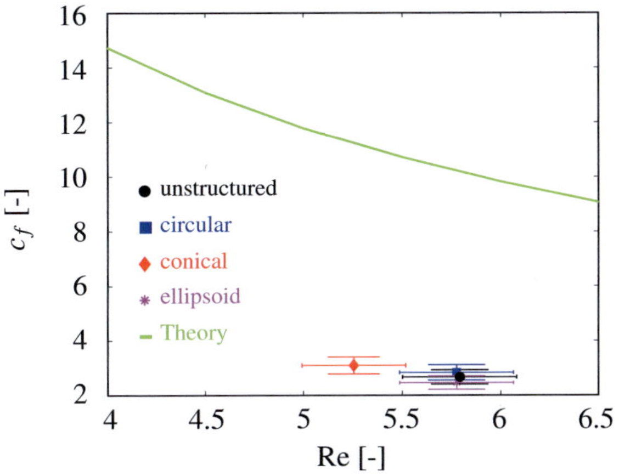

Figure 4.8.: Nikuradse diagram calculated from the μAPTV results.[81]

is brought into the Wenzel state during the μAPTV measurements. This transition could be triggered by the motion of the fluid and the occurring pressure gradient between the air-liquid interface. This could lead to a decrease of the amount of entrapped air and even a complete wetting of the surface. Secondly, if the fluid is already in the Wenzel state, the shape of the surface structures will greatly influence the fluid behavior, because they lead to higher friction and disturbances of the flow at the wall.

Table 4.3.: Results of the dynamic contact angle measurements showing the receding contact angle (rec. CA), the advancing CA (adv. CA) and the contact angle hysteresis (CAH).

identification	rec. CA [°]	adv. CA [°]	CAH [°]
unstructured	56.4 ± 0.17	79.5 ± 2.34	23.1
circular structures	67.4 ± 4.29	103.1 ± 9.61	35.7
conical structures	75.4 ± 5.66	101.8 ± 3.95	26.4
ellipsoid structures	61.7 ± 1	87.3 ± 1.1	25.6

4.3. Further Applications in Medicine

Micro- and nanostructured surfaces are also highly interesting for applications in medicine, because they can influence tissue-implant interactions as well as fluid behavior. In this work the fabrication of medical equipment was examined. First, small tubes with structures on the inside and outside were produced, leading to different surface properties due to the structuring. These tubes allow an *in vitro* analysis of fluids as well as tissue behavior and show the chances of microtechnology for medical applications. Afterwards, a micropipette with structured surfaces was fabricated, showing the easy fabrication of tubes with different diameters.

Micro- and nanostructures on surfaces can improve biocompatibility of implants. Rough surfaces, with $R_z > 100\,\mu m$ lead to a good incorporation into the surrounding tissue and is used for long-term implants. A medium roughness leads to a reversible incorporation into the tissue and is therefore utilized for temporary implants. Implants with a roughness of $R_z < 0.1\,\mu m$ do not support tissue growth and finds applications in cardiac valve prostheses. Commonly, the surface roughness of metallic implants is adapted to an application. Especially the surfaces of brain implants are thoroughly adjusted. The material is not allowed to move within the brain tissue but on the other hand should also not lead to excessive cell growth.[8]

Because of the inexpensiveness and mass fabrication capabilities polymeric products are often used in medicine for disposable products like catheters. Catheter is the generic term for a tubular device, which is inserted into the body through vessels or body cavities for diagnostic or therapeutic purposes. The most common infection associated with catheters are urinary track infections and blood stream infections due to venous catheters. These nosocomial infections are a high risk to patients because around two thirds of all hospital patients receive a venous catheter.[89]

4.3.1. Tubes

Micro- and nanostructured surfaces can help increase biocompatibility and time of usage. The objective of this work was to examine fabrication methods that allow the production of tubes with different structures on the inside and outside. This is necessary to satisfy the different demands, like for example, prohibiting cell proliferation of venous cathers. Additionally, structures prohibiting back flow as well as supporting a complete emptying of the tube can also be benefical for catheters.

In this work, tubes with structures on the inside and outside were fabricated.[90] First double-sided hot embossing was utilized to structure a thin foil on both sides with different structures. Afterwards, a tube was formed by twin-sheet forming. The structures on the inside of the channel show a superhydrophobic behavior, while the structures on the outside lead to a controlled tissue behavior. A SEM micrograph of the tube is shown in Figure 4.9. These tubes can be utilized as venous catheters or as prototypes for testing new surface structures *in vitro*.

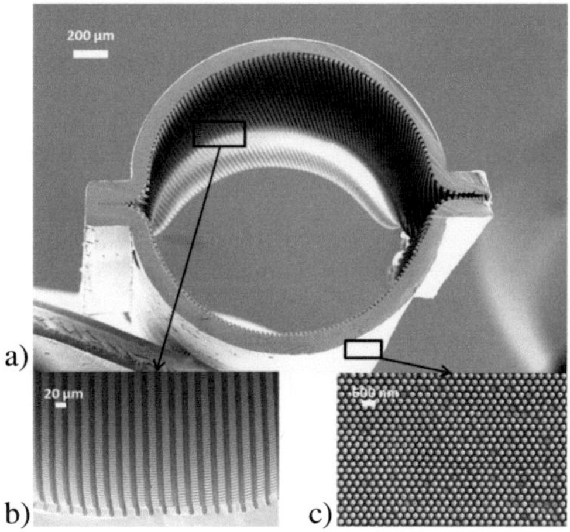

Figure 4.9.: SEM micrographs of a) a tube after removing the residual layer with b) microstructures on the inside and c) nanostructures on the outside.[90]

Hot embossing and microthermoforming, commonly creates a residual layer. In this work a hot cutting method was introduced to remove this residual layer. A schematic view of the setup is shown in Figure 4.10. This process allows the separation of parts from their residual layer and, additionally, improves the bond strength, due to a welding of the two foils at the bonded area. A heating element is embedded into a metal block with connected blades. The tube with the residual layer is placed in a positioning tool. The blades are heated by the heating element to a temperature around the glass transition temperature of the material. The material is then cut and melted at the same time. By melting the material at the cutting area the two foils are welded together leading to a higher bond strength.

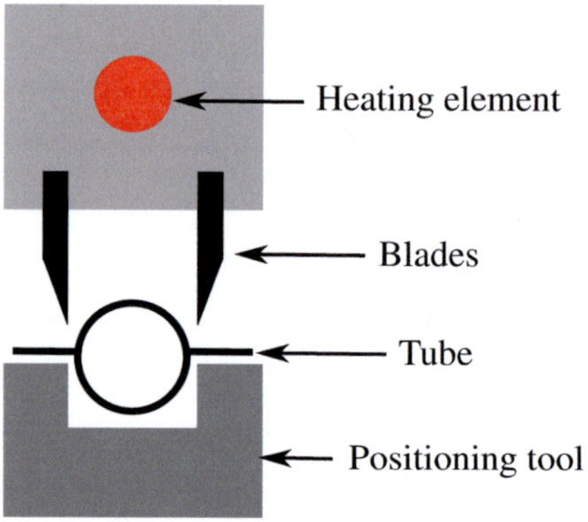

Figure 4.10.: Schematic view of the hot cutting mechanism. The tube with the residual layer is placed into a positioning tool. Blades are heated over a heating element to the glass transition temperature and pressed down, cutting and melting the residual layer at the same time, leading to a separated tube with welded bond areas.[90]

4.3.2. Micropipette

Another objective was to fabricate pipettes, with micro- or nanostructures on the inside, that assure a complete emptying of the pipette. Therefore, micropipettes with a length of 40 mm and an outer diameter of 400 μm, 800 μm and 2 mm were fabricated. An image of the fabricated micropipette can be found in Figure 4.11. The pipette is structured with nanostructures on the inside to avoid depositions and assure a complete emptying of the pipette. The nanostructures reflect the light depending on its angle of incidents, which leads to the different colors on the micropipette image. A two-step process, combining hot embossing and twin-sheet forming, was utilized to fabricate these parts.

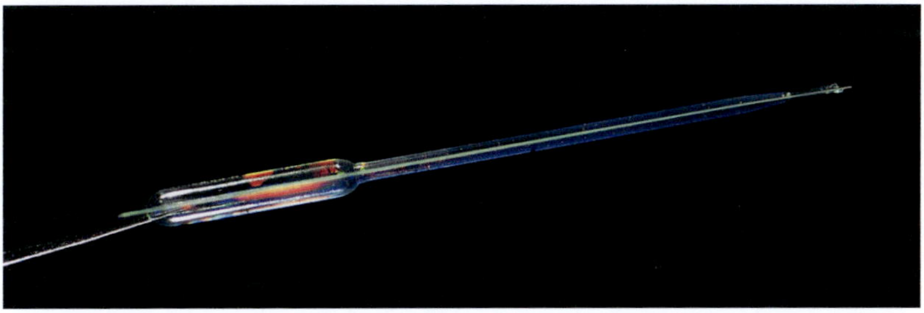

Figure 4.11.: Micropipette with a length of 40 mm and outher diameters of 2 mm, 800 μm and 400 μm. Nanostructures on the inside lead to a superhydrophobic surface to avoid depositions inside the pipette as well as to assure a complete emptying of the pipette.

4.4. Conclusion and Outlook

In this chapter the static fluid behavior was first analyzed by contact angle measurements. A dependency of the contact angle on the material was shown as well as the increase of the contact angle due to surface structures. Hydrophilic materials were successfully brought into the hydrophobic regime by surface structures, enabling the fabrication of microfluidic devices with controlled fluid behavior.

Afterwards, the dynamic fluid behavior was examined by micro astigmatism particle tracking velocimetry. This method utilizes particles to image the velocity profile of a fluid. Three differently structured channels were utilized as well as an unstructured channel. A change in velocity was observed and, by calculating the Darcy friction factor and the Reynolds number from the measured data, the friction of these channels could be compared.

When comparing contact angle measurements and μAPTV measurements no apparent correlation can be found. One possible explanation is, that the influence of the dimensions of the structures and their air retaining capabilities has more influence on the fluid behavior than the contact angle hysteresis. To allow predictions about the fluid behavior on the basis of contact angle measurements, further experiments are necessary. Pressure loss experiments could give information about losses inside a microchannel as well as about the wetting behavior under flow conditions. A new set of experiments to determine friction, as well as the state of the fluid, needs to be conducted. In these experiments the pressure loss between two points inside a microchannel should be measured, enabling the calculation of the Fanning friction factor. This is necessary, because both the friction factor and the Reynolds number are highly dependent on the dimensions of the channel. If the fluid is in the Cassie-Baxter state, higher Fanning friction factors are measured because of a smaller effective channel height and width. This leads to a distortion of the real effects inside the channel. Figure 4.12 shows a depiction of a fluid in the Cassie-Baxter state and in the Wenzel state and the effective height of the channel. Therefore, the experiments should be conducted with water and another liquid with a low surface tension (e.g. silicone oil). A low surface tension would lead to a complete wetting of the surface and therefore the Wenzel state. The gained results can than be compared to experiments with water and conclusions about the wetting behavior can be made.

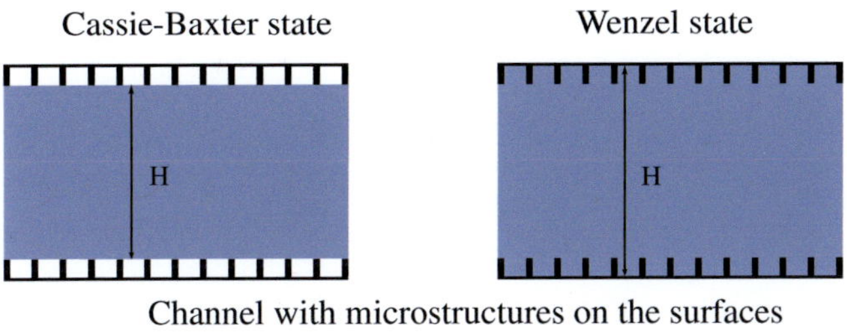

Figure 4.12.: Fluid in the Cassie-Baxter state and Wenzel state and effective height of the channel.

At the end of this chapter, two applications for structured surfaces influencing fluid behavior as well as tissue-surface interactions are introduced. First, tubes with different structures on the inside and outside were produced. Secondly, micropipettes with varying diameters and structured surfaces were fabricated. Both devices can be used for *in vitro* experiments to analyze tissue-surface interactions as well as flow behavior. A possible application for these devices are in medicine as catheters. Because the length of the devices is limited by the size of the mold inserts, catheters fabricated by hot embossing and microthermoforming can only find an application as venous catheters or as winged infusion sets. However, the findings gained from *in vitro* testing can be used to define structure dimensions for different applications. To fabricate long catheters, as needed for different applications (e.g. urinary catheters), extrusion would be an interesting fabrication process. This process is capable of continuous production of tubes and by adapting parts of the extrusion setup, would be capable of fabricating structured tubes.

5. Proteinadsorption

Thermoplastic materials entered the field of medicine and biology in the 1960s.[8] They were mainly used as disposables, like catheters and syringes and lead to a significant decrease of infections. They are also gaining more and more attention due to their inexpensive and fast fabrication. Today, they are not only used for diagnostic purposes but also for long-term implants like cardiac valves. Additionally, they are often found in tissue engineering or utilized for drug delivery systems. However, a drawback of thermoplastic materials is the unspecific adsorption of biomolecules. This could for instance lead to biofilm formation on surfaces[91] or to a poor signal-to-noise ratio in diagnostic tools. Therefore, laborious surface treatments are necessary to inhibit and control the adsorption of biomolecules on thermoplastic surfaces.[92,93,94] Unfortunately, these surface modifications can not be integrated in a mass fabrication process and therefore only a few microfluidic Lab-on-a-Chip devices are established on the market. To address this, a new method for locally controlled biomolecule adsorption is presented by micro- and nanostructuring surfaces. The structuring leads to a superhydrophobic surface and a fluid in the Cassie-Baxter state. This surface is characterized by a three-phase interface between liquid, surface structures and trapped air, causing a favored biomolecule adsorption on this interface. To confirm this theory, protein adsorption on different micro- and sub-micrometer structures was analyzed for fluorescence labeled bovine serum albumin and streptavidin.[95]

Afterwards this new method of biomolecule adsorption is utilized to detect the c-reactive protein based on a clinical procedure.[96] Experiments in buffer solution as well as in human serum were conducted, showing the ability to distinguish different antigen concentrations. The proposed prototype is fully capable of being integrated into mass fabrication by hot embossing or injection molding.

5.1. Laser Scanning and Fluorescence Microscopy

Fluorescence microscopy is a common method to analyze biological samples. The setup is comparable to a standard optical microscope. The sample is illuminated by monochromatic light of a specific wavelength, absorbed by the fluorophore and re-emitted as fluorescence at a different wavelength. This fluorescence light is collected in an objective, passes through an emission filter and is then observable through the ocular or by a camera. Two commonly utilized fluorophores are fluorescein isothiocyanate (FITC) and Texas Red. The excitation for FITC (and its derivative AlexaFluor 488) is at 497 nm (blue) and the emission at 520 nm (green). For Texas Red the excitation is at 589 nm (yellow) and emission at 615 nm (orange). Because excitation and emission are close together, it is very important to confine the excitation wavelength to a narrow band to avoid unspecific fluorescence. Sometimes the excitation and emission curves overlap, which can lead to a re-absorption of the emitted light. Also the autofluorescence of the surrounding materials at a specific wavelength should be measured for quantitative analysis. Additionally, the fluorescence intensity is in general very low, leading to a poor signal-to-noise ratio and difficult interpretation of the data. The fluorescence intensity further decreases with continuos illumination, due to photobleaching. Besides photobleaching, concentration quenching can also lead to an decrease in fluorescence intensity. For low concentrations an increase in fluorophore concentration leads to an increase in fluorescence intensity, while higher concentrations of fluorophore can decrease the intensity. Also an uneven illumination can produce to false results.[97,98]

Additionally, stray light can lead to halo-like effects in fluorescence images. To avoid these, confocal laser scanning microscopy (CLSM) can be used to increase the spatial resolution. In these microscopes the area of excitation as well as the area of emission is confined to a small three-dimensional pixel called voxel. This spot is scanned over the specimen leading to a high resolution image with a low amount of background fluorescence, stray light and noise. Due to its high resolution in the z-direction it is also possible to generate three-dimensional images. This makes it very popular in biology, especially for cell observation.[97,98]

5.2. Localized Protein Immobilization

Two proteins, bovine serum albumin (BSA) and streptavidin were utilized for adsorption experiments on structured surfaces. BSA is commonly used for passivating surfaces. This protein easily adsorbs on surfaces and therefore inhibits the adsorption of other proteins in these areas. Streptavidin is often used because of its high affinity to bind biotin. The streptavidin-biotin bond is one of the most popular methods for non-convalent conjugations and is commonly used for immunoassays. Each streptavidin molecule contains four binding sites for biotin and its strong interaction makes it very useful for assays and specific targeting applications. This bond is also very stable even under extreme conditions like variations in buffer salt concentration, pH, change in temperature or in the presence of denaturants or detergents.[99]

5.2.1. Experimental Setup

The experiments are divided into two sets. In the first set, the proposed immobilization method is verified. The second set works with different buffer solutions and pH-values to examine the influence of buffer solution on adsorption behavior. All experiments were first conducted with BSA and afterwards with streptavidin. BSA was purchase from Life Technologies and labeled with the fluorescein AlexaFluor 488 (Excitation 497 nm Emission: 520 nm) with 7 mol of AlexaFluor 488 per mol BSA. Streptavidin was purchased from Sigma-Aldrich marked with 3-9 mol FITC per mol streptavidin with the same excitation and emission peak wavelength than the FITC derivative AlexaFluor 488.

To examine the influence of the buffer agent three different buffers were used. A potassium hydrogen phthalate (PHP) buffer with a pH-value of 4.0 (CAS-Number: 877-24-7), a phosphate buffered saline (PBS) solution with a pH-value of 7.4 (0.01 M phosphate buffer, 0.0027 M potassium chloride, 0.137 M sodium chloride in 200 ml deionized water), and a 50 mM Tris-borate buffer (Tris) with a pH-value of 8.

The structured Polysulfon (PSU) and Cyclic Olefin Copolymer (COC) foils were fabricated by hot embossing. For most experiments the polymer foil was sealed to the base plate by a PDMS (Polydimethylsiloxan) foil to achieve a liquid tight channel. The sealing was reversible and the PDMS-foil as well as the base plate were reused after being cleaned by Ethanol and Isopropanol. Laser welding was also examined for the fabrication of the channels, because of its mass fabrication capabilities (see Chapter 3).

The fabricated channel was filled with a mixture of buffer agent and protein solution by pipetting the mixture into the channel inlets. For BSA and streptavidin a concentration of 0.0625 μg/μl was utilized. This solution was incubated at room temperature for three hours. During incubation the fluid in- and outlets were sealed with tape to avoid evaporation or contamination. Afterwards the channel was rinsed by the buffer, dried and examined under a fluorescence microscope. For the fluorescence analysis a Nikon TI-E fluorescence microscope was used. A schematic view of the experimental procedure is shown in Figure 5.1. The fluorescence images were examined by the software "ImageJ".

First channels with the developed layout were utilized. The channels were structured with six fields with round pillars with a height of approx.

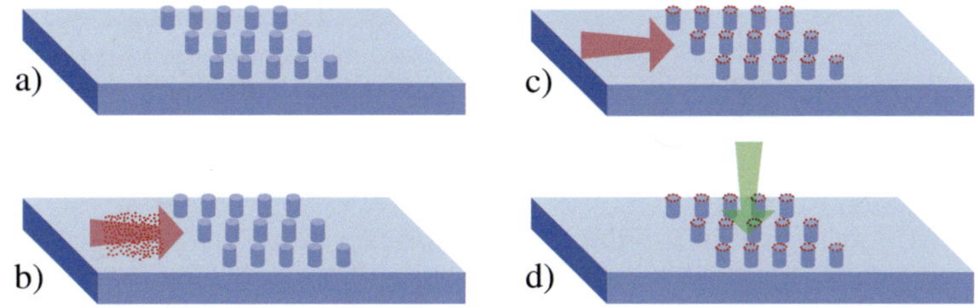

Figure 5.1.: Schematic view of the experimental procedure. a) A channel is structured on at least one sidewall an b) incubated with a protein and buffer agent for three hours. c) The channel is rinsed and dried and d) examined with a fluorescence microscope.

85 µm and a diameter of 10 µm, 15 µm, 20 µm, 25 µm, 30 µm, and 35 µm. The pitch was 4·Ø.

Additionally, the experiments were repeated with structures with diameters of 500 nm, 750 nm and 1 µm and a pitch of 2·Ø. The height of the structures was approx. 900 nm. All experiments were conducted with BSA as well as with streptavidin. Afterwards all experiments were repeated with different buffer solutions.

After adsorption experiments also the desorption was examined. First BSA was adsorbed on the surface as described before and afterwards a 1 % sodium dodecyl sulphate (SDS) - water solution was incubated for three hours. The channel was then rinsed, dried and analyzed by fluorescence imaging.

5.2.2. Results

First the adsorption on the developed design was analyzed. After rinsing and drying, the samples were examined with a fluorescence microscope. Clear and dominant rings with a high intensity were observed. The larger rings had the same diameter as the microstructures. The width of the larger rings was dependent on the diameter of the pillars. For a diameter of 35 µm the width was between 5 µm and 3.5 µm. An additional smaller ring, inside of the larger ring, was also observed and diameters of 12.5 μm ± 0.5 μm were measured. The width of these smaller rings was below 2 μm. The intensity of the pillar top is in general higher than the intensity of the background. Therefore the pillars are clearly distinguishable. Figure 5.2 shows an SEM micrograph of a pillar and the corresponding fluorescence image with intensity profile.

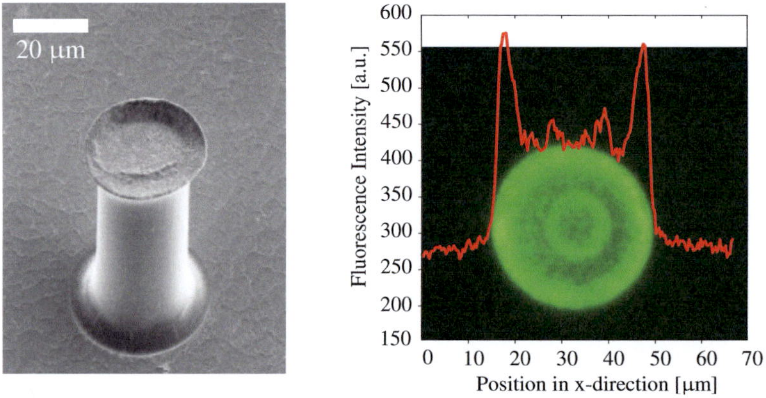

Figure 5.2.: SEM micrograph of a pillar with a diameter of 35 μm and a height of 85 μm and a fluorescence image (Top view) of the same pillar with its intensity profile. The fluorescence image shows a clear ring of high intensity on the edge of the pillar. An additional smaller ring of high intensity is observed in the middle of the pillar.

The larger outer ring of high fluorescence intensity can be explained by a preferred protein adsorption on the edge of the pillar. This would be in good agreement with the proposed theory. The proteins are moving to the air-liquid-solid interface at the edge of the pillar, and immobilize there through physical adsorption. The second smaller ring can be explained by molding defects. The SEM micrograph shows a curved edge of the pillar giving it a cup-like appearance. The size of the second ring corresponds to the size of the cup-bottom. Therefore, it is assumed that at this location further interfaces arise because of a change in shape. Another explanation for the ring like structures can be optical effects. The different reflective indices of air and the polymer can lead to a reflection on the air-solid interface. This reflection can take place either between the pillars or inside of the material. The rate of reflection is very small, leading to a negligible impact of this factor. Additionally, total internal reflexion on the edge of the pillar could be possible, leading to a whispering-gallery mode like behavior.[100] This behavior is only possible if the circumference of the ring is exactly a multitude of the wavelength, which is not the case for the proposed pillars. This effect also needs very sharp edges, because every defect leads to light scattering on the interface. Another possibility is a signal enhancement due to protein adsorption on the whole pillar. Adsorption on the whole pillar would be possible for a totally wetted surface. The increase in surface area would lead to higher fluorescence intensities. This effect was used by Zhang et al[101] to enhance the fluorescence intensity of a photonic crystal biosensor by structuring the surface with nanorods. Because of the measured contact angles an adsorption on the whole pillar is not possible. Another optical effect is diffraction. Diffraction is wavelength dependable and can easily be excluded by repeating the experiments with proteins labeled with different fluorophores. Experiments with a TexasRed labeled biomolecule showed similar results. Therefore, diffraction is not possible.

To examine the position of the proteins on the pillar, confocal laser scanning microscopy was used to achieve a high resolution in z-direction. Images were taken in 1.5 µm steps from the top of the pillar towards the bottom. The voxel size was 0.07 µm x 0.07 µm x 1.5 µm. An excerpt of these images are shown in Figure 5.3. The fluorescence intensity shows in some fluorescence images an almost even intensity distribution over the top of the pillar but still with a slightly higher intensity at the edge of it. While getting downwards fading fluorescence is observable on the pillar for around 20-25 µm. Afterwards as well as on the bottom of the pillar and on the foil no fluorescence is observed. The slowly decreasing fluorescence intensity is assumed to be due to light scattering. In conjunction with the results of the contact angle measurements for these structures it is shown, that the protein adsorption only takes place on top of the pillar with preferred adsorption on the edge of the pillar.

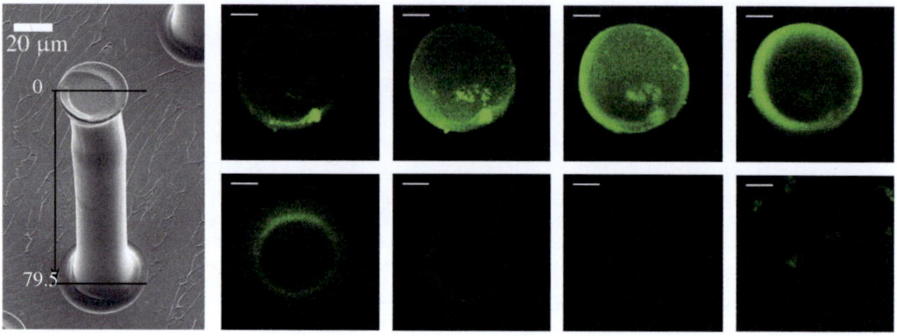

Figure 5.3.: SEM micrograph of a pillar with a diameter of 20 μm and a height of approx. 85 μm. On the right a series of images taken with a laser scanning microscope. First four images show slices of the top of the pillar in 1.5 μm steps. Second row shows images after 9.5 μm, 19.5 μm, 30 μm and 79.5 μm from the first image. Scale bar is 5 μm in the fluorescence images.

When using structures of 1 μm and less also rings of higher fluorescence intensities are observed. For pillars with a diameter of 500 nm and a pitch of 1 μm, individual pillars are no longer distinguishable from each other, because of the limitations in resolution of the microscope. Therefore, intensity measurements were taken from unstructured and structured areas. This enabled the analysis of the fluorescence intensity due to the structures in comparison to unstructured areas. A photograph of the foil with corresponding SEM micrographs of the three examined fields and fluorescence images of these fields are shown in Figure 5.4. The fluorescence images also show an uneven distribution of the fluorescence. In Field 1 and 2 larger defects are visible. These defects are mostly because of imperfections in the mold insert or from contaminations during hot embossing, leading to an incomplete filling of the mold cavities. Additionally, as can be observed in Field 3, accumulations of proteins can occur.

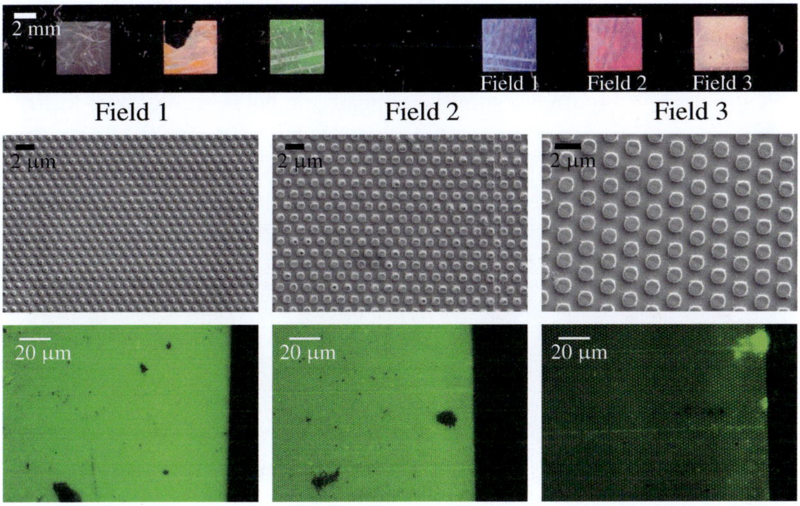

Figure 5.4.: Photography of the foil with different structured fields and their corresponding SEM images as well as fluorescence images with AlexaFluor 488 labeled BSA. Field 1 is structured with cylindrical pillars with a diameter of 500 nm, Field 2 with a diameter of 750 nm and Field 3 with a diamter of 1 μm, a pitch of twice the diameter and a height of approx. 900 nm.

The second set of experiments analyzed the influence of the buffer agent on the adsorption properties. The used fluorophore AlexaFluor 488 has a constant fluorescence intensity for pH-values between 4 and 10.[102] Therefore, the fluorescence intensity for the different buffer solution can be compared. A distinct difference in intensity can be observed depending on the buffer agent and therefore the pH-value. For BSA the highest fluorescence intensity and therefore the highest adsorption was present for PHP with a pH-value of 4. This is in good agreement with the literature, because of the isoelectric point (pI) of BSA, which is at 4.6.[103] The pI is the pH-value at which the protein has no net electric charge,[14] which means, that the total charges inside a protein cancel each other out, leading to an electrical neutral molecule. Because of this neutrality the repulsion between two proteins is negligible and higher packing densities of the proteins per area are possible.[104] Furthermore, because the electric charges cancel each other out, the net intramolecular Coloumb force is attractive, leading to a compact protein structure.[20] Figure 5.5 shows a comparison between the three utilized buffer agents.

35 μm

10 μm

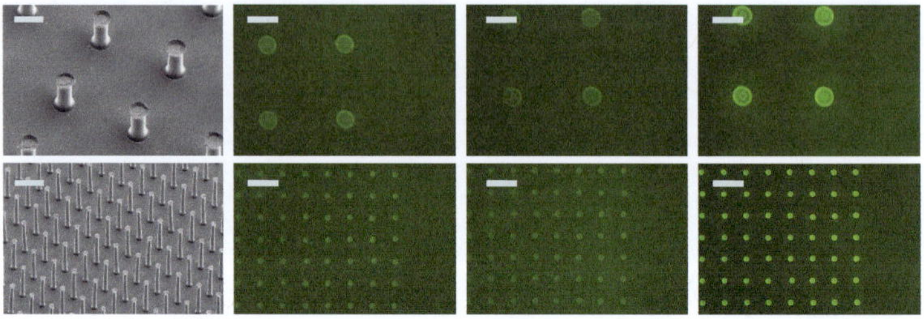

SEM micrographs   Tris-borat pH = 8   PBS pH = 7.4   PHP pH = 4

Figure 5.5.: Left: SEM micrographs of hot pulled micropillars with a diameter of (upper row) 35 μm and (lower row) 10 μm, a height of approx. 85 μm and corresponding fluorescence images with different buffer agents. Scale bar: 50 μm.

Because BSA is known to readily adsorb on surface, all experiments are repeated with streptavidin. Figure 5.6 shows a SEM micrograph of a pillar with a diameter of 20 μm and a height of 85 μm. As observed before with BSA, ring-like structures appear with the same outer diameter and shape as the pillar. While the fluorescence intensity for PBS is low, there is no difference for Tris and PHP. The utilized fluorescence label FITC has a strong dependency on the pH-value. For pH-values greater 7 the intensity increases. This could lead to the contradictory findings. The high intensity at a pH of 4 is due to a higher adsorption of streptavidin, while the high intensity at a pH of 8 is due to the intensity increase due to the pH-value.[102] A comparison with the pI of streptavidin is not possible, because multiple pI for streptavidin are known and the supplier also only provides a multitude of pI-values for this protein. Additionally, the labeling of streptavidin with

FITC was compared to BSA very low, which lead to a poor signal-to-noise ratio.

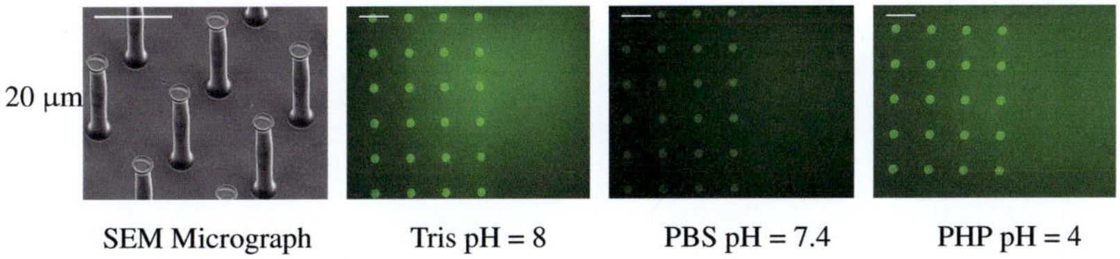

Figure 5.6.: Results of streptavidin adsorption experiments on hot pulled surfaces. Left: SEM micrograph of hot pulled micropillars with a diameter of 20 µm and a height of approx. 85 µm. On the right corresponding fluorescence images with different buffer agents. Scale bar: 50 µm

Desorption experiments of proteins with 1 % SDS were conducted. Figure 5.7 shows the absolute fluorescence intensity before and after desorption as well as the background fluorescence of the material. Again, depending on the buffer solution higher or lower decreases of fluorescence intensities were observed. Depending on the pH-value even an increase in intensity was possible. For PSU an increase of fluorescence intensity was measured when using PHP as a buffer solution. When comparing pre- and post-desorption images, an even distribution of the fluorescence is observed compared to the pre-desorption images. Molding defects and aggregations are no longer visible. This can be explained by the properties of SDS. SDS is a surfactant and leads to a decrease in surface tension of a fluid followed by a complete wetting of the surface. Proteins are then unfolded by the surfactant and solubilized. Additionally, the buffer solution will also lead to a change of electrical charge on the surface. This electrical charge can induce a re-adsorption and higher affinity of already adsorbed proteins. The fluorescence images in Figure 5.8 show an example for PSU on Field 3 before and after desorption.

Additionally, all experiments with structures of less than 1 µm were repeated with Cyclic Olefin Copolymer. The results were similar to PSU but

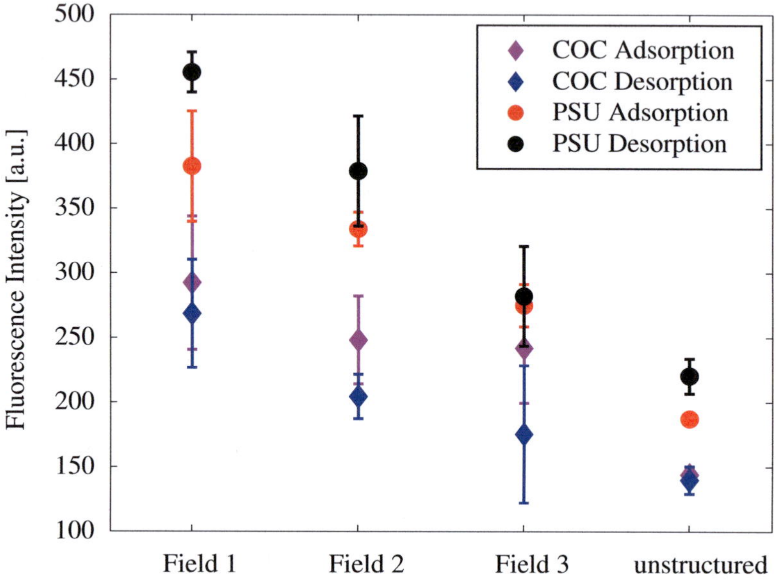

Figure 5.7.: Comparison of fluorescence intensities after adsorption and after desorption of BSA on PSU and COC with PHP as a buffer solution.

a) 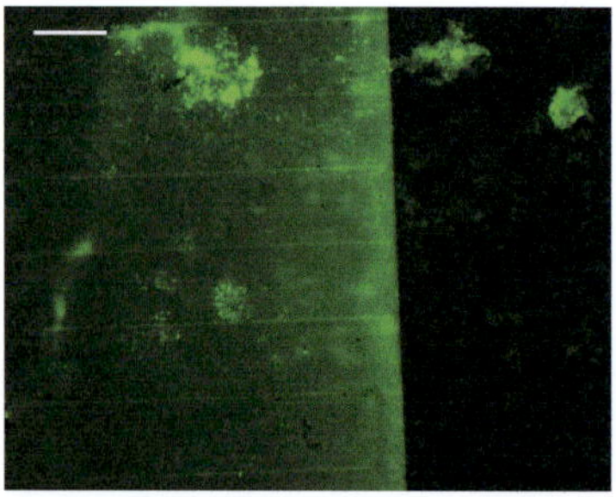 b) 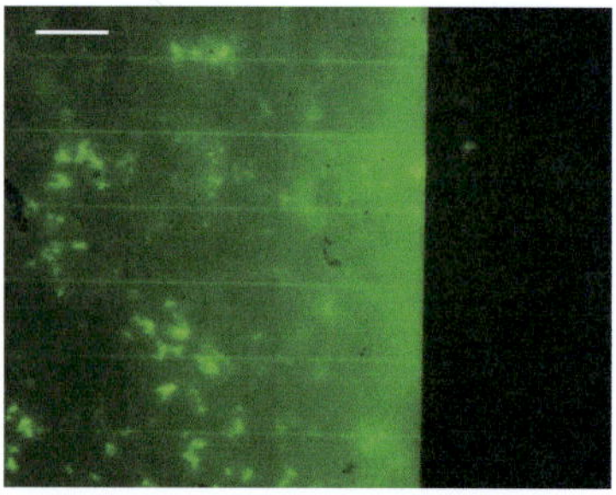

Figure 5.8.: Fluorescence image after a) adsorption and b) desorption of BSA on PSU on Field 3. Accumulations of proteins are visible. The proteins are solubilized and re-adsorb all over the material, because of the low surface tension, the fluid is no longer in the Cassie-Baxter state and the material is completely wetted. Scale bar: 50 µm.

the fluorescence intensity was for Tris and PBS generally higher. This could be due to the optical properties of the material or due to the pH-value of the buffer solution. Depending on the buffer solution the surface charges of the material can change, leading to an increase or decrease in protein adsorption. A comparison of COC and PSU for different buffer solutions is shown in Figure 5.9. The experiments are shown for structures with a diameter of 500 nm and a pitch of 1 μm. These structures show the highest sensitivity due to their large circumference to area ratio. The y-axis shows the ratio of the fluorescence intensity of the structured areas to the unstructured areas of the material.

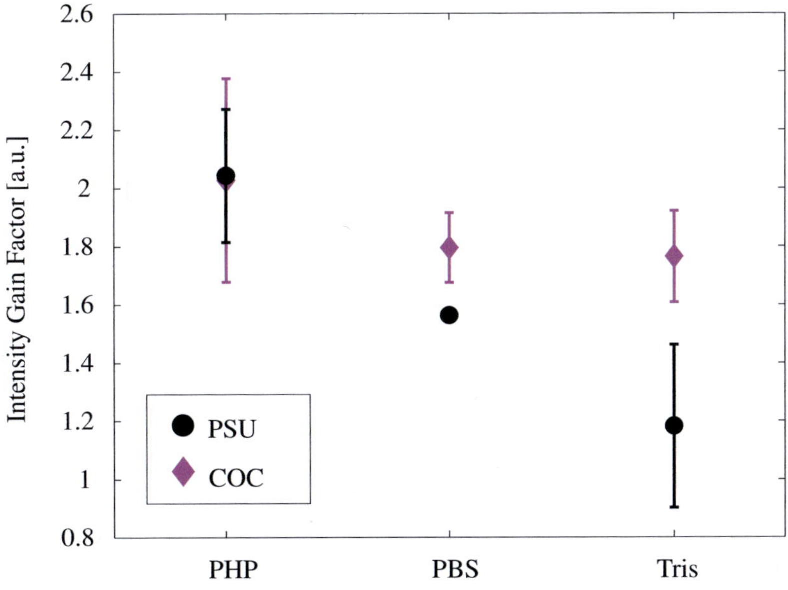

Figure 5.9.: Comparison of adsorbed BSA on COC and PSU on structures with a diameter of 500 nm and a pitch of 1 μm for the three buffer solutions PHP, PBS and Tris.

5.3. Sandwich-Assays

Sandwich-Assays belong to the group of immunoassays, like enzyme-linked immunosorbent assays (ELISA) and lateral flow assays. These biochemical tests analyze the presence and concentration of biomolecules in a solution by binding a specific biomolecule to an antibody. They are used for diagnostic procedures in medicine and biology and consist of immobilized biorecognition elements, like enzymes, antibodies, etc. A well known example for a lateral flow assay is the home pregnancy test.

When using an ELISA or lateral flow assay, different biosensor principles are available to conduct the experiment. Biosensors consist of a biorecognition element, determining the selectivity of the sensor, and a transducer element. The transducer transforms a biological or biochemical reaction into an output signal and determines the sensitivity of the sensor. Biosensors are classified by their transducer into five groups:[105]

- Electrochemical
- Optical
- Acoustic or gravimetric
- Thermal or calorimetric
- Magnetic

In this work a new optical biosensor, based on structured surfaces, was developed.[44] In the following section the developed transducer principle is tested in different environments. Preliminary tests were conducted to analyze the possibility of streptavidin-biotin bonds. Afterwards sandwich-assays for the detection of c-reactive proteins in buffer as well as in human serum are conducted.

5.3.1. State of the Art

Two groups of optical biosensors are known, with label and label-free. Labels are typically fluorophores, nanoparticles or carbon nanotubes.[106,105] These labels are bound to biorecognition molecules or target molecules[107] and can be excited either by light, chemically or electrochemically.[105] Each time light of a specific wavelength is emitted.

Label-free detection methods utilize refraction. The most common method is surface plasmon resonance (SPR) introduced in 1983 by Liedberg et al.[108] SPR can be used on metal surfaces, covered by a dielectric. When excited by light at a resonance wavelength, an electromagnetic wave propagates along the metal-dielectric interface due to total internal reflection. This leads to an evanescent wave. Once molecules adsorb on the surface the propagating wave is disturbed and light is emitted. Difficulties of these method is the coupling of the light into the system. This is in general done by prisms, waveguides, optical fibers or gratings.[107,109] Also common for biosensing are interferometers like the Mach-Zehnder interferometer or the Young interferometer. These sensors consist of one waveguide that is split into two. One of these waveguides is open to the surrounding and the evanescent wave can interact with the environment. When the two waveguides recombine the resulting interference can be measured by a photodetector. Another label-free sensing methods are optical ring resonators, photonic crystals or Bragg gratings. Optical ring resonator utilize the whispering gallery effect.[100] A ring-like structure is fabricated and light is coupled into the structures. The light propagates through the material by total internal reflection until molecules bind to the structure. Photonic crystals consist of periodic domains of low and high diffractive indices. Depending on the wavelength evanescent waves can travel through them until molecules adsorb on the surface. Bragg gratings work on a similar principle. In general the light is trapped inside the grating but when distorted the light propagates and can be detected.

5.3.2. Experimental Setup

When proteins adsorb on surfaces the conformation of the protein can change. This can lead to a loss in binding sites or denaturation. Therefore, the first set of experiments was to examine these effects by utilizing a sandwich-assay, which could be utilized to detect a DNA mutation leading to cystic fibrosis disease. First streptavidin was immobilized on the structured surface. Unconjugated streptavidin was purchase at Biomol and was used in a concentration of 0.1 mg/ml. Afterwards, the system was incubated with BSA at a concentration of 0.125 mg/ml. BSA was used to block free binding sites on the surface. In the last step, a biotinylated DNA string with a Texas Red fluorescence marker was incubated in the channel. The DNA string had 18 base pairs, with the sequence 5' –TAG AAA AAA GTT GGA TCC –3' pairs which are the complementary base pairs to the DNA mutation leading to the disease. This oligonucleotide was purchased from Purimex and was used in a concentration of 0.2 nmol/µl. A schematic view of the experiment is shown in Figure 5.10. Incubation was 2 hours for each process step.

After the preliminary experiments a sandwich-assay for the detection of c-reactive protein (CRP) was conducted. CRP is an acute phase protein synthesized by the liver during an inflammation.[110] Depending on the grade of inflammation the CRP concentration in the blood is changing. For a healthy body the CRP concentration is below 10 µg/ml. When a severe inflammation is present concentrations of over 500 µg/ml are possible. In the conducted experiments concentrations of 1 µg/ml, 10 µg/ml and 100 µg/ml were used as well as a blank sample. These experiments were first conducted in PBS as a buffer solution. Afterwards the experiments were repeated in human serum.

For the detection of CRP, first streptavidin was immobilized on the surface. Afterwards a biotinylated CRP-antibody (concentration 0.2 µg/µl) was incubated, binding to streptavidin via a streptavidin-biotin bond. Afterwards BSA was incubated and used to block free binding sites on the polymer surface to avoid binding of the antigen or the secondary antibody onto the surface. Then the analyte, a mixture of buffer agent or human serum and CRP binds via the lock-key principle to its antibody. In the last step another CRP-antibody with a fluorescence marker (FITC) in a concentration of 0.5 μg/μl binds again via the key-lock principle with the CRP. Every biomolecule was incubated in the microchannel for 2 hours and the channel was rinsed with buffer solution before the next biomolecule was brought into the channel. At the end the channel is rinsed, dried and examined with a fluorescence microscope.[96] A schematic view of the different layers of biomolecules is shown in Figure 5.11.

CRP was purchased from Biotrend. Biotinylated and FITC-labeled anti-CRP as well as unconjugated streptavidin was purchased from Biomol. The

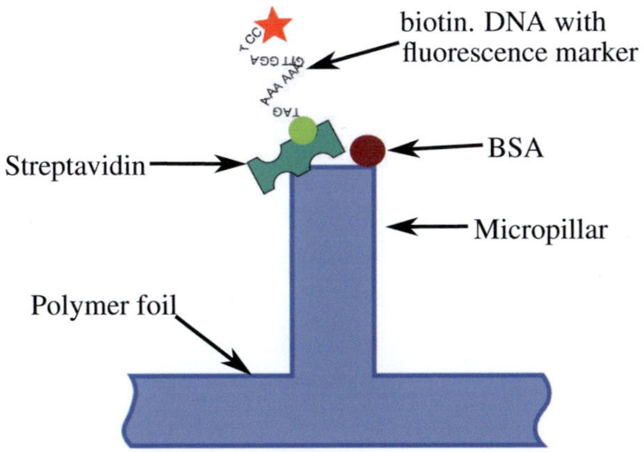

Figure 5.10.: Preliminary experiment to examine functionality of adsorbed proteins. First streptavidin is immobilized on a surface. Afterwards BSA was used to block free binding sites. Then a biotinylated DNA string with a Texas Red fluorescence marker is joined with streptavidin via a streptavidin-biotin bond.

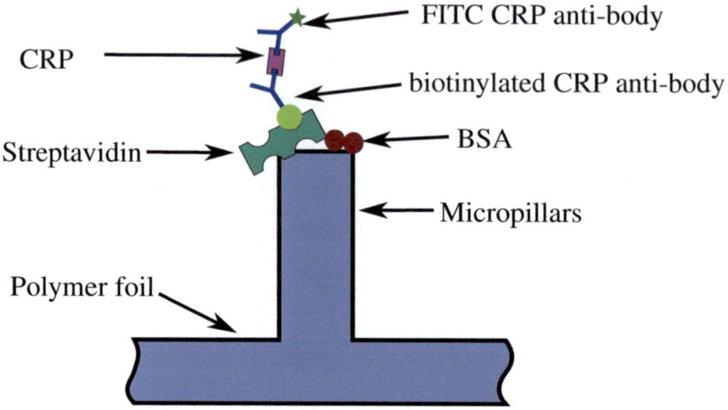

Figure 5.11.: Experimental setup for the detection of CRP. First Streptavidin is immobilized on the surface, afterwards a biotinylated antibody is bound to the streptavidin. BSA is then incubated to block free binding sites. Afterwards CRP in buffer solution or human serum is brought onto the surface and binds to the anti-CRP. In the last step a FITC labeled CRP antibody is bound to the CRP.

lyophilized biomolecules were re-hydrated with deionized water or buffer solution.

For all experiments nanostructured foils (as seen in Figure 5.4) with three fields were utilized (Field 1 having a diameter of 500 nm, Field 2 of 750 nm and Field 3 1 μm). These experiments were also used to evaluate the sensitivity of the sensor. The fluorescence intensity is dependent on the number of adsorbed proteins, which in turn is dependent on the available binding sites. For the utilized foil the ratio of pillar top to area is for all fields 20 %, because the pitch is a multiple of the diameter. When analyzing an elementary cell with a size of 6 μm x 6 μm, the circumference in contrast doubles from the smallest structures (500 nm in diameter) to the larger structures (1 μm in diameter). If the adsorption of the proteins would be linear with the available area, the fluorescence intensities for Field 1 should be twice as high as the fluorescence intensity of Field 3. A summary of the geometric properties is given in Table 5.1.

Table 5.1.: Geometric properties (Dieamter (D), Pitch (P), Height (H), Elements per EC (EEC) and Circumference in EC (CEC)) of the used nanostructured foil. With the size of an elementary cell (EC) of 6 µm x 6 µm.

	D	P	H	EEC	$\frac{A_{PillarTop}}{A_{EC}}$	CEC
Field 1	500 nm	1 µm	900 nm	36	19.63 %	56.55 µm
Field 2	750 nm	1.5 µm	900 nm	16	19.63 %	37.7 µm
Field 3	1 µm	2 µm	900 nm	9	19.63 %	28.27 µm

For analysis fluorescence images were taken showing a structured and unstructured area. These images have the advantage, that the unstructured area is giving a measurement of the background fluorescence of the image. Because the fluorescence microscope had an uneven illumination, images of unstructured areas were taken to flatten the images and avoid false results. These background images were averaged and to reduce noise, large defects were flatten by a median filter. This filter averages one pixel by taking into account the surrounding pixels. After this, an average background image was obtained and used as a reference. Every fluorescence image was than divided pixel by pixel with the average background image. Figure 5.12 shows an image before flattening and after flattening and its fluorescence intensity profile.

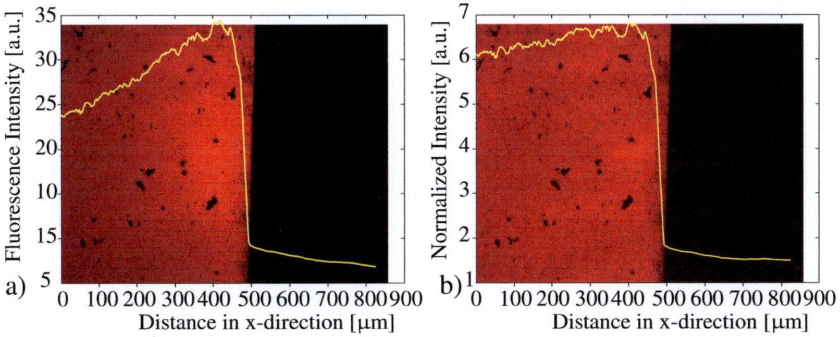

Figure 5.12.: Fluorescence images and intensity profiles a) before normalizing and b) after normalizing it to the background image.

Afterwards the mean normalized fluorescence intensity for the structured area and the unstructured area was calculated as well as the standard deviation. The standard deviation was not utilized for further calculations. But it gives important information about the quality of the structuring by hot embossing. Three measurements per field and sample where taken while three experiments with the same setup were conducted leading to nine mean fluorescence intensities per experiment. Again the mean value and the standard deviation of these nine values were calculated and divided with the mean value of the blank unstructured sample. This leads to the intensity gain factor (IGF) (Eq. 5.1), which is used to describe the results.

$$IGF = \frac{I_{meanStructureSample}}{I_{meanUnstructuredBlank}} \tag{5.1}$$

5.3.3. Results

The first experiments analyze the functionality of streptavidin after adsorption on the surface. Figure 5.13 shows the results of these experiments. Black icons show the unstructured areas of the blank samples and magenta diamonds show the structured area. Blue circles represent the unstructured areas of samples with immobilized streptavidin, BSA and bound DNA, where a small increase in fluorescence intensity compared to the blank sample is already observed. Red diamonds indicate the structured areas with the complete assay (streptavidin-BSA-DNA), which intensity is 6 times higher than for the assay on the unstructured area. This enhancement in intensity can greatly improve the sensitivity of a sensor.

In theory, the intensity of Field 1 should be twice the intensity of Field 3. In this graph, the intensity increase from Field 3 to Field 1 is approx. 1.7. These experiments also show, that the sensitivity of the sensor can be tuned by the dimensions of the structures on the surface. These experiments also showed, that the physical adsorption of streptavidin leaves enough binding

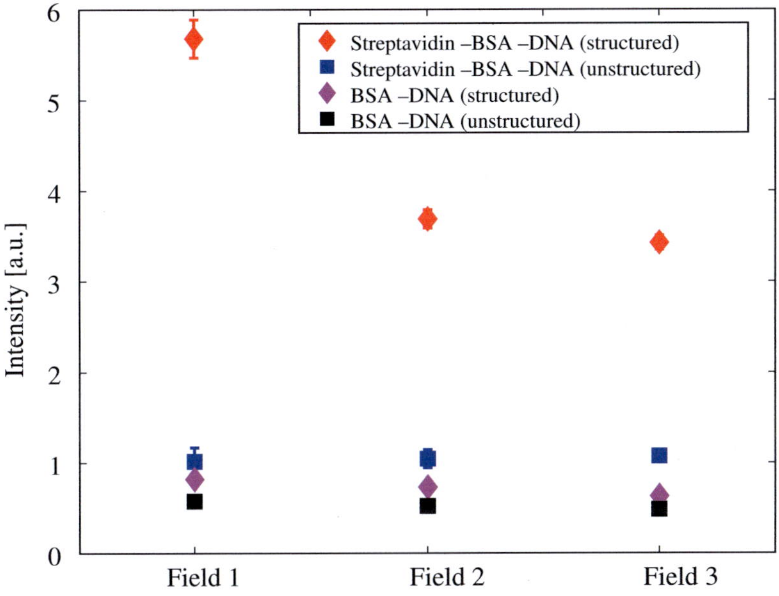

Figure 5.13.: Intensity of the blank sample unstructured areas (black blocks), structured areas (magenta diamonds) and the sample on the unstructured areas (blue blocks) and structured areas (red diamonds). The graph shows a distinct increase of the intensity by structuring a polymer foil. The errorbars are given as ± standard deviation.

sites to successfully perform streptavidin-biotin bonds. Additionally, it can be assumed that no denaturation took place.

Afterwards sandwich-assays for the detection of CRP were conducted. First PBS was used as a buffer solution. The results in Figure 5.14 show a clear distinction between the blank sample, the clinical threshold 10 μg/ml and 100 μg/ml.

Additionally, these experiments were repeated with human serum as a buffer agent. Human serum is the liquid part of blood without cellular molecules, like red blood cells, and it contains therefore a multitude of proteins, vitamins, enzymes etc. When using human serum, typically matrix

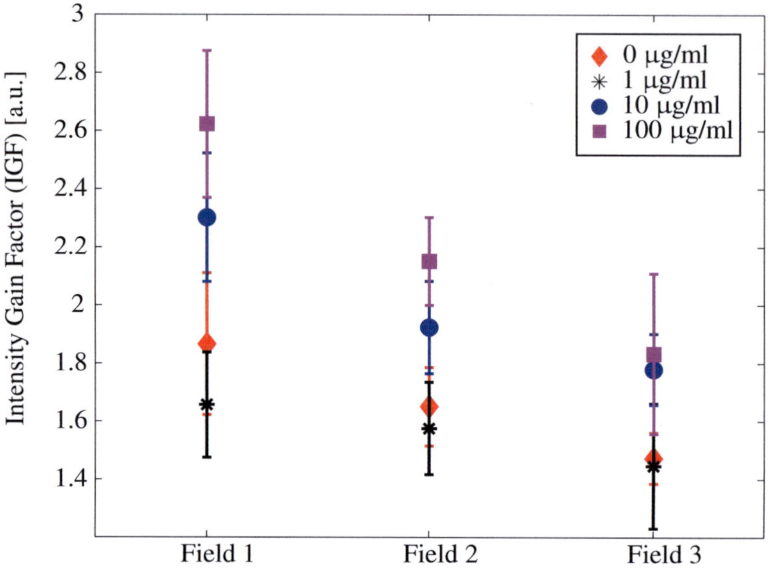

Figure 5.14.: Results of sandwich assays for the detection of CRP in PBS. The errorbars are given as ± standard deviation.

effects due to the multitude of biomolecules in the serum are observed, leading to a poor signal-to-noise ratio. These effects are not observed in this work. A clear distinction between the different concentration is shown in Figure 5.15. While a high intensity gain factor increase is found for 1 μg/ml to 10 μg/ml, the intensity gain factor increase between 10 μg/ml and 100 μg/ml is smaller. This could be due to concentration quenching. In clinical diagnostic procedures it is common to dilute the blood sample to avoid matrix effects. When diluting the sample, less concentration quenching will take place, which would even increase sensitivity of the introduced sensor.

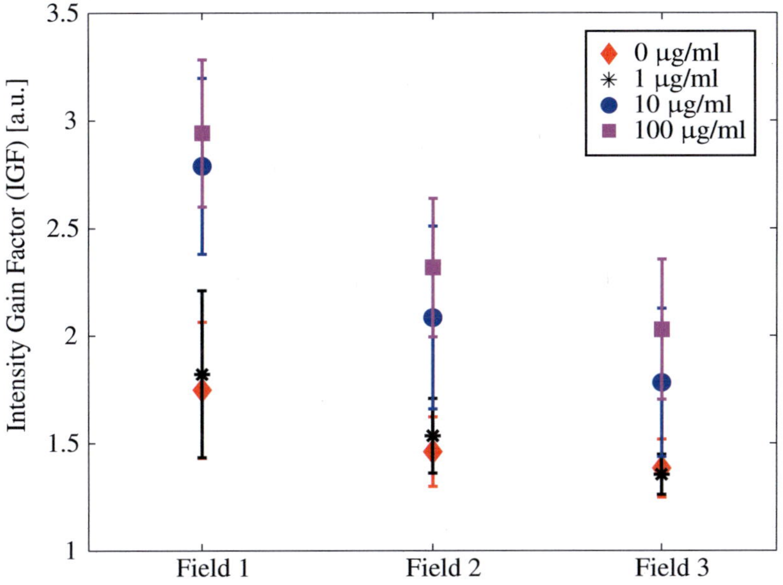

Figure 5.15.: Results of CRP in human serum

5.4. Conclusion

This work introduced a promising new method for protein adsorption on micro- and nanostructured surfaces. The structuring of the surface lead to a fluid behavior in the Cassie-Baxter state, which in turn promoted a preferred protein immobilization on the structure edges. This was confirmed by confocal laser scanning microscopy, showing the highest fluorescence intensity on the edge of the pillar. Imaging the sidewalls of the pillars a decreasing fluorescence intensity is observed in the first few micrometers, because of light scattering.

For all experiments, cylindrical pillars with a circular cross section were utilized. But also other shapes would be possible and could influence the adsorption rate. Öner and McCarthy[42] discussed the influence of structure shape (e.g. rhombus, star, indented square) on the wetting behavior. When using such shapes, the water is pinned to the surface, which leads to higher contact angles. In this work it was observed, that higher adsorption of proteins was achieved on the edge of defects. Therefore, other shapes could lead to higher protein adsorption rates.

Structures with diameters of 1 µm and less were also analyzed. These structures showed high fluorescence intensities on structured areas compared to unstructured areas. Different buffer agents lead to an increase or decrease in adsorption rate depending on the isoelectric point of the used protein. Additionally desorption experiments showed that proteins can be desorbed from the surface using SDS.

Streptavidin was immobilized on the surface without denaturation or loss of binding sites. This was confirmed in sandwich-assay utilizing a biotinylated DNA. This preliminary test can also be used to detect a disease called cystic fibrosis disease, by using the described biotinylated DNA without a fluorescent label. After introducing an analyte with the complementary DNA into the microfluidic chip, it binds to the biotinylated DNA and can be detected by fluorescent labeling. Afterwards sandwich-assays for the detection of c-reactive proteins were utilized to test the proposed transducer method. Different concentrations of c-reactive protein in buffer as well as in human serum were successfully measured. It was possible to precisely distinguish between blank samples and the clinical threshold of 10 µg/ml, as well as other concentrations. Further optimization is necessary to bring this product closer to the market. Especially the length of the experiment needs to be reduced. Therefore, the adsorption rate over time should be analyzed to decrease the incubation times of the different steps. Additionally, other proteins for blocking free binding sites need to be tested to achieve better blocking. This can significantly increase the signal-to-noise ratio and lead to better results.

For Point-of-Care diagnostics, disposable products and portable devices are necessary. This product already showed its capabilities for mass fabrication and, therefore, as a product for single usage. The cooperation part-

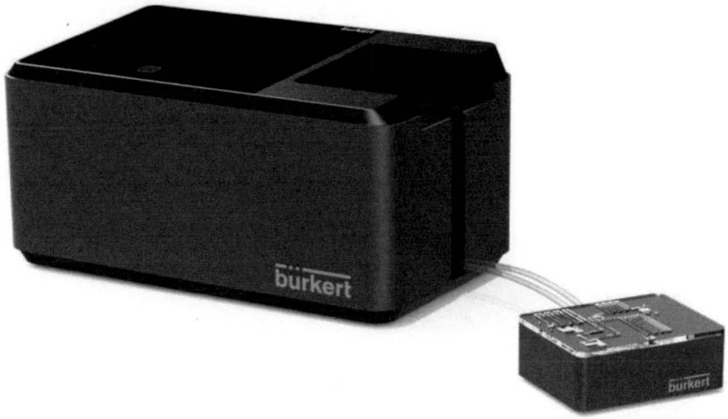

Figure 5.16.: Portable read-out device for the Lab-on-a-Chip system developed by Bürkert Fluid Control Systems.[111]

ner Bürkert Fluid Control Systems developed a portable device (see Figure 5.16) for the introduced Lab-on-a-Chip system.[111] This device consists of syringe-pumps, with an accuracy of 1 µl, a temperature control unit, a LED-diode and a photo-detector with a sensitivity of 1 ng/µl in ambient light or of less than 0.1 ng/µl in darkness. The portable device also contains a display, connected to a processing unit, to analyze and visualize the results immediately. This portable device, in combination with the introduced immobilization method, can be used for immunoassays directly at the patient. Because of the inexpensive Lab-on-a-Chip design and the easy handling, this could also find an application in areas of conflict or third world countries.

6. Cell Experiments

Defined areas of protein immobilization are also of great interest for cell experiments, because proteins are utilized to define areas of cell growth. Therefore, the introduced immobilization method of a preferred protein adsorption on structured surfaces is utilized to examine cell growth.

To analyze the biological response of cells, experiments with single cells are of high interest. Often structural traps are utilized to separate and trap cells, like microwells[112,113] or cell trapping arrays.[114,115] Additionally dielectrophoresis is used to guide cells by applying a heterogeneous electric field. Cells are then transported away or towards dense electrical fields depending on the dielectric properties of the cells and the surrounding medium. This method can be used for cell trapping[116] and even cell patterning.[117]

Furthermore, the topography of a surface greatly influences the proliferation, size, alignment, motion and adhesion of cells.[118,119] Klein *et al.*[120,121] fabricated three-dimensional scaffolds by direct laser writing to achieve free hanging cells. First microposts with connecting beams were produced from PEG-DA (Polyethylene glycol diacrylate) to inhibit cell attachment, in a second direct laser writing step, small Ormocomp squares were fabricated, allowing cell growth on these squares. The fabricated microposts were additionally utilized to examine cell forces applied on the posts.[120,122] Fu *et al.*[123] used microposts to influence cell morphology, adhesion and stem cell differentiation. A few applications in medicine already use roughened surfaces to enhance biocompatibility of implants.[8] By working with defined geometrical structures, new and interesting applications arise. Especially biologist are very interested in these structures to analyze the behavior of cells and gain new insights into differentiation and proliferation.

In first experiments, in cooperation with the Bioanalytics group of Prof. Petra Dittrich at the ETH Zürich, the biocompatibility of different polymeric materials was analyzed. Afterwards cell growth and behavior experiments were conducted on various structured surfaces. These experiments enabled a precise design of new layouts for further cell experiments.

6.1. Basic Principles

6.1.1. Cells

Cells are defined as "The basic unit from which living organisms are made, consisting of an aqueous solution of organic molecules enclosed by a membrane. All cells arise from existing cells, usually by a process of division".[124] Two main classes of cells are known, prokaryotic and eukaryotic cells. Prokaryotic cells, like bacteria, are the most basic cells. Eukaryotic cells are assumed to have evolved from prokaryotic cells and are much more complex. Eukaryotic cells are the basic module for fungi, plants and animals.[125] These two classes share the same genetic code, metabolic pathways, plasma membrane, etc. But cells in general differ greatly in size, design, function and behavior. Cell sizes can range from a few micrometers up to 1 millimeter in length. Small cell sizes are often found in bacteria like the Bdellovibrio bacteriovorus,[125] which is less than 5 µm in length and approx. 500 nm in width, while a frog's egg is 1 mm in diameter.[124] The design of a cell is greatly depending on its surrounding and function. While for example nerve cells are extremely extended with large branching to receive signals from up to 100.000 other cells, muscle cells in contrast need a stiff substrate and will grow tightly to it in a fibrous manner.

6.1.2. Cell Culture Substrates

Two types of cell culture substrates are available. The traditional flat, two-dimensional (2D) cell substrates and the newly emerging three-dimensional (3D) substrates. 2D substrates are usually made out of glass or polystyrene (PS). Glass was originally used for cell cultures because of its easy sterilization, satisfactory optical properties and surface charge.[126] Electrostatic forces in combination with van-der-Waals-forces are the greatest influence factor on cell adhesion.[127] Important charge carrier are bivalent cations and proteins. Inadequate cell adhesion on a substrate will lead to inhibited cell proliferation. In recent years, PS became the most common 2D substrate. The advantages are an inexpensive manufacturing and therefore disposable substrates, and good optical properties. It is commercially available as flask, petri dishes or multiwell plates. But PS is a hydrophobic material, which does not support cell proliferation. This leads to pre-treatment of the surfaces by various methods like, corona discharge, gamma-irradiation or chemical treatments.[126,127] 2D culture substrates are capable of cell proliferation in a monolayer. This approach is often criticized, because it does not accurately reproduce physiology.[128] Therefore, 3D cell substrates were introduced to reproduce the extracellular matrix (ECM) in tissue. The space between cells in tissue is filled with the ECM and it provides structural support, e.g. help maintain the shape under physical loads or gravity.[129] The ECM also supports biochemical functions[129,130] and determines the shape and behavior of the cell.[125,126,130] To reproduce the ECM different synthetic and natural materials are available.[126,131] These materials are brought into a three dimensional matrix by electrospinning, gas foaming, dry freezing, printing techniques, etc.[131]

6.1.3. Sterilization

Contamination of cell cultures can effect the cells greatly. Cell growth can be inhibited, the production of cell-products can be reduced and even death and therefore destruction of the cell culture is possible.[132] Because decontamination of a cell culture is very difficult or even impossible, sterilization of culture substrates as well as of equipment is mandatory. Sterilization methods are divided into four groups: sterilization by heat, chemical sterilization, irradiation, and filters.

Sterilization by Heat

Heat is the most common method for sterilization. It is well known from the food industry, where pasteurization is a typical method for sterilization. Pasteurization uses low temperatures between 55-60 °C for many hours. While bacteria and viruses are inactivated at temperatures of 60-80 °C, spore-forming bacteria and prions are more resistant and need higher temperatures or different approaches. A standard process is autoclaving. This process utilized pressurized steam and temperatures of 121 °C to sterilized surfaces. When using dry heat, temperatures between 160 °C and 180 °C as well as longer cycle times are necessary. But when working with thermoplastic polymers, high temperatures can affect polymer structure.[8,132]

Chemical Sterilization

Chemical sterilization is commonly used for syringes and filters, and can be divided into fumigation and liquid disinfectants. Different gases can be used for fumigation like ethylene oxide, hydrogen peroxide or formaldehyde. Ethylene oxide has the strongest sterilization properties but gets absorbed by the material.[8] This absorption leads to long venting times to deabsorbe the material again. This is important because ethylene oxide is also toxic for cells. Hydrogen peroxide is utilized at low temperatures and leads to 90% shorter cycle times than sterilization by ethylene oxide. Formaldehyde gas is commonly used to sterilize airflow cabinets or rooms for cell handling.

Liquid disinfectants, like aldehydes, hypochlorite, phenolics or alcohol, are often used on equipment and surfaces. The disinfectant is applied by spraying, wiping with a cloth or towel, or immersion of the equipment inside a container of disinfectant. Alcohol, like ethanol or propanol, is the least effective disinfectant and is typically utilized for surfaces and gloved hands.[132]

Irradiation

Materials that cannot be treated by heat or chemically, are sterilized by irradiation. When sterilizing rooms or culture cabinets, ultraviolet irradiation at a wavelength of 254 nm[8] is utilized. This method is capable to inactivate microorganisms and viruses but, due to is poor penetration power, only on surfaces. This problem is overcome by using gamma rays. Typically a dose of 25kGy from a cobalt-60 source is utilized. Because of its great penetration, equipment that is already packed and sealed can be sterilized.

6.2. Experimental Setup

To analyze different structures and their use in cell proliferation, two cell lines were utilized. The first cell line, C2C12, is a mouse myoblast cell, first introduced by Yaffe and Saxe.[133] These cells are capable of proliferation and differentiation in cell culture and are adherent cells, which form fibers. The second cell type is a canine kidney cell line, called Madin-Darby Canine Kidney Cells (MDCK), named after Madin and Darby.[134] These cells form a monolayer when growing and are commonly used to study cell growth *in vitro*.

At the beginning of the experiments the thermoplastic polymer foils were sterilized, by rinsing the samples with ethanol. Afterwards the surface was covered with fibronectin, a protein involved in different cellular interactions like cell growth, adhesion, migration and differentiation.[135] Cells in a cell culture medium were then placed on the foil and incubated. Afterwards the cell membranes were dyed and analyzed with a fluorescence microscope.

The first experiments were to analyze PSU and COC for their biocompatibility. MDCK and C2C12 cell lines were incubated on these thermoplastic foils and examined after one and four days. The second set of experiments analyzed the impact of structures with a diameter of 1 μm, 750 nm and 500 nm on C2C12 cells. Structures with a height of 85 μm and diameters ranging from 10 μm to 35 μm were utilized for the third set of experiments to examine cell sorting capabilities, by defining areas of high protein concentration. These areas of high protein concentration are on top of the pillar and should lead to a preferred cell growth in these areas. For these experiments MDCK and C2C12 cell lines were utilized. The fourth set of experiments was aimed to analyze cell stretching capabilities. Therefore, the micropillars on these foils have a constant pitch, but their size is constantly decreasing, leading to a decrease in distance. Again, MDCK and C2C12 cells were used for this set of experiments. The different materials as well as the different designs are shown in Table 6.1 and Figure 6.1.

Table 6.1.: Geometrical properties of the used polymer foils for cell experiments.

Layout	Material	Diameter [μm]	Pitch	Height [μm]
Fig.6.1 a	PSU, COC	0.5, 0.75, 1	$p = n \cdot d$ with n=2..5	1
Fig.6.1 b	PSU	10 - 35	$p = 4 \cdot d$	85
Fig.6.1 c	PC	45 - 1	p = 45 μm	1.5

6.3. Results and Discussion

The first experiment was to analyze cell growth on PSU and COC foils. As a reference the cells were placed on the thermoplastic material and a standard PS well plate for cell experiments. After 24 hours of incubation the cells were examined under the microscope. There was no visible distinction between the different substrates. Figure 6.2 shows images after

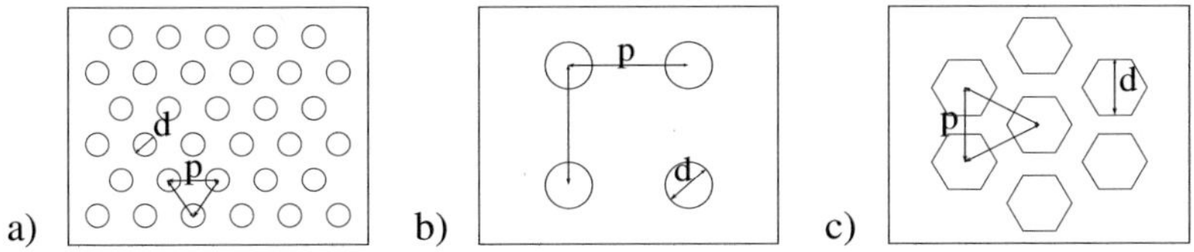

Figure 6.1.: Layout of samples for a) second set of experiments, b) third set of experiments and c) fourth set of experiments.

24 hours and after 96 hours for MDCK and C2C12 cell lines on COC and the well plate. Cell growth on PSU was identical to the COC foil and PS well plate and is therefore not shown.

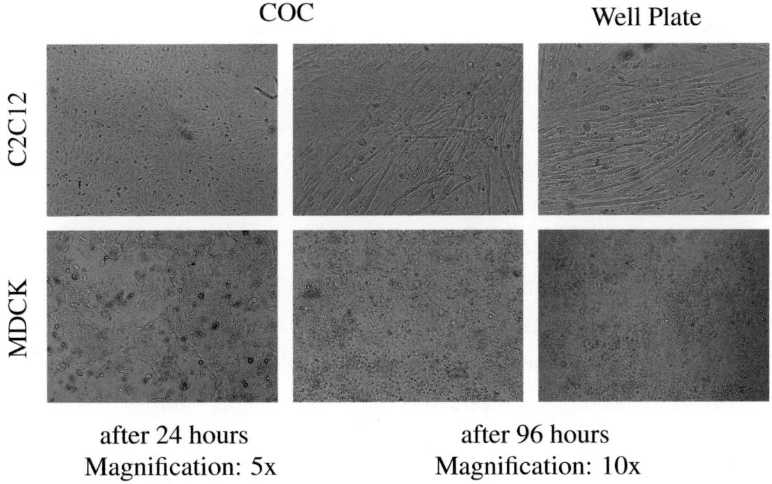

Figure 6.2.: MDCK and C2C12 cell growth on a COC foil and a standard PS well plate after 24 and 96 hours.

The next set of experiments was to analyze cell growth in comparison with protein adsorption experiments. In theory, proteins should adhere in areas with a high protein concentration. Fluorescence images were taken of unstructured areas, structured areas as well as images showing both areas.

The cell shape on all areas did not differ from each other. This is valid for both cell lines on COC and PSU. Figure 6.3 shows fluorescence images of C2C12 cells growing on unstructured and structured areas (pillar diameter 500 nm).

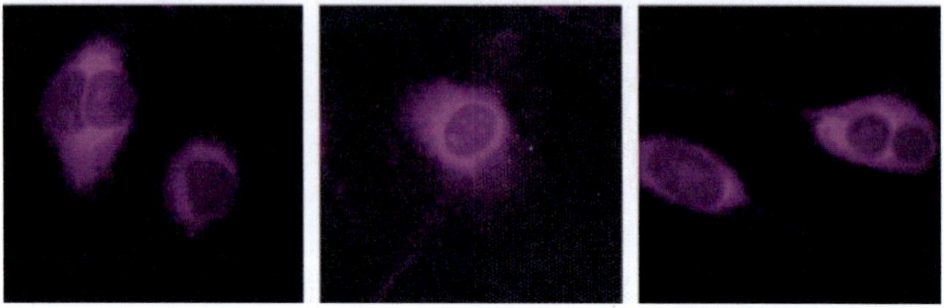

Figure 6.3.: Fluorescence image of a cell growing on unstructured areas, the boundary between unstructured and structured areas as well as on structured areas. The fluorescence is due to a membrane dye. Magnification: 64 times.

In the third set of experiments the possibility of cell separation was analyzed, by adhesion of a single cell on one micropillar. Experiments showed, that while some cells adhered at the top of the pillar, most cells were growing between the pillars on the foil. When assuming, that the fluid is in the Cassie-Baxter state, this is not possible, because cells cannot survive outside of the culture medium. Therefore, the experimental procedure was examined. To avoid contamination of the surface the sample was first sterilized with ethanol and without a drying process fibronectin was placed on the foil. Due to the small surface tension of ethanol a complete wetting of the surface took place. This in turn was followed by a complete wetting with fibronectin and the culture medium. This lead to an even cell growth on structured and unstructured areas in the second set of experiments. To avoid these a different experimental procedure is necessary.

In the last set of experiments a similar cell growth than in set two and three was observed. Again, because of a complete wetting of the surface, the whole substrate was covered in fibronectin and, therefore, the cells did not distinguish between pillar and surface, this was also supported by the small height of the pillars.

6.4. Conclusion and Outlook

Thermoplastic polymer surfaces are well suited for cell experiments and tissue engineering. The growth on thermoplastic polymer with, and without structures did not differ from growth on standard cell well plates or glass substrates. This opens a wide field of applications. Depending on the cell type and desired proliferation, a matching thermoplastic polymer can be chosen, especially in regard of the Young's modulus.

When using thermoplastic materials only a few sterilization methods are possible. Autoclaving at 121 °C was first utilized. This lead to swelling of the material and destruction of the structures due to water absorption. Afterwards ethanol was used for sterilization. Ethanol in turn is lowering the surface tension of the material, leading to a hydrophilic surface and therefore the Wenzel-state. For further experiments, gamma ray irradiation is recommended.

In this work further experiments were designed. First the cell separation by micropillars was revised. The new layout of the substrates consists of microposts, with diameters of 1.5 times the size of the used cell and an aspect ratio of 2. This should give enough space to enable a good adhesion on the surface as well as cell growth. This could also lead to a fast and inexpensive possibility to separate cells and conduct single cell experiments.

But when separating cells on one pillar, another interesting question arises. Do cells overgrow pillars? When a cell reaches the edge of the pillar, will the cell grow down or just stop growing? How far can and do cells stretch to reach the next pillar? For these experiments, pillars with a height of twice the cell's diameter, a pillar diameter of half the cells size and a slowly increasing distance should allow interesting insights into the cell stretching behavior. By having slightly smaller pillars than the size of cell should assure the necessity of the cell to stretch to the next pillar. This can enable to identify a critical distance between pillars, which cells cannot overcome. This distance can then be implemented into the cell separation layout.

Surfaces with micropillars can also be used to measure exerted forces of the cell on a surface by the bending angle of the pillars. Currently, these experiments are conducted with micropillars fabricated from PDMS.[136, 137] PDMS is a very flexible material, which yields and in turn leads to a distortion of the results. By using polymeric materials, the Young's modulus can be determined accurately and lead to higher force resolutions.

Additionally, experiments to control cell growth along a path of proteins should be continued. After changing the experimental protocol, especially the sterilization process, a stable Cassie-Baxter state should be possible. Therefore, a localized protein immobilization on the pillar edges as shown in Chapter 5 should be reproducible. This enables the analysis of protein growth and movement along a given path due to the proteins.

7. Conclusion and Outlook

While miniaturized system are already a part of our daily life, they are still underrepresented in the important field of medicine, biology and life-sciences. Especially, the lack of an inexpensive fabrication procedure often hinders products to enter into the market.

This work presented a new method to immobilize biomolecules on thermoplastic materials without laborious surface modification by utilizing the preferred movement and adsorption on interfaces. Therefore, artificial interfaces were created by influencing the fluid behavior into the Cassie-Baxter state. In this state air is trapped between structures on the surface, leading to a three-phase interface at the edge of the structures.

To bring this design closer to the market, different fabrication methods were utilized, all capable of mass fabrication. A combination of hot embossing and micro injection molding was discussed as the most promising and inexpensive process for the fabrication. Additionally, the combination of hot embossing, microthermoforming and bonding enabled the production of fully structured, three-dimensional microfluidic systems.

These fully structured microfluidic devices enabled the analysis of the fluid behavior in dependency of the surface structures. Contact angle measurements showed a change in wetting behavior in dependency of the surface structures and material. Additional dynamic measurements by micro astigmatism particle tracking velocimetry gave information about the fluid behavior in a flow, showing a reduced friction depending on the surface structures. This also enables the production of channels with a passive fluid control. By alternating hydrophilic and superhydrophobic areas, passive valves can be achieved, which can be controlled by the fluid pressure. The proposed combination of fabrication methods also allowed the production of medical equipment like catheters and micropipettes. By structuring the inside and outside of tubes, the fluid behavior on the inside can be controlled, as well as the tissue-surface interactions. This can lead to a better biocompatibility and longer dwell time.

After establishing a mass production capable fabrication process, the proposed design was examined for its protein immobilization capabilities. Experiments with BSA as well as streptavidin showed a preferred adsorption on interfaces, observable by clear ring-like fluorescence intensity profiles of the size of a micropillar. A clear dependency on material as well as on buffer solution was also observable. Experiments showing no denaturation or loss of function of streptavidin were conducted with a sandwich-assay for the detection of a DNA mutation leading to cystic fibrosis disease. Afterwards, this immobilization method was utilized to detect c-reactive proteins in buffer solution as well as in serum. The concentration of this protein indicates an inflammation as well as the severity of it. A clear distinction between the critical value and the blank sample was possible as well as a distinction between different concentration in buffer solution as well as in human serum.

Different micro- and nanostructured polymer foils were utilized for cell experiments at the ETH Zürich. A very good biocompatibility was observed for the used thermoplastic polymer foils. Cell proliferation experiments enabled the development of new designs. These new designs can lead to a new method for cell separation as well as give information about cell stretching capabilities.

Furthermore, optimization of the proposed sandwich-assay could increase sensitivity and decrease the length of diagnosis. Further experiments about the adsorption behavior on polymeric surfaces can lead to an optimized buffer solution and thermoplastic material to achieve high adsorption rates and increase therefore the sensitivity of the sensor. The sensitivity can also be increased by an adjusted micro- or nanopillar design. Additionally, different blocking agents than the utilized BSA can lead to higher signal-to-noise ratios. Furthermore, experiments analyzing the adsorption rate over time are interesting to optimize incubation times and therefore the overall length of diagnosis.

Additionally by combining lithographic methods with the proposed immobilization method, a fast, maskless, and cheap method to achieve covalent immobilization is possible.

During this work, Bürkert Fluid Control Systems GmbH developed a prototype for a portable read-out device for the introduced microfluidic chip. This device consists of syringe pumps, light source, a photo-detector and hard- and software for analysis. The software can analyze the fluorescence intensity in-process and present the results on an incorporated display.

The combination of different fabrication methods as well as the utilization of physical effects lead to a microfluidic chip, capable of mass fabrication. The introduced immobilization method is easy to use, robust and reproducible. This microfluidic chip can be used in combination with a portable device, for Point-of-Care diagnostics. Because of the easy handling it can also be used in areas of conflicts and by untrained personnel.

A. List of Publications

A.1. Patents

1. N. E. Steidle, T. Hahn. *Nanostrukturen/Bioreaktionen*, German Patent Application: DE 102013111759. (2013)

A.2. Articles

1. N.E. Steidle, T. Hahn, C. Bader, M. Schneider, R. Ahrens, M. Worgull and A.E. Guber. *Micro- and nanostructured microfluidic chip for specific protein immobilization*, Proceedings of the 17th International Conference on Miniaturized Systems for Chemistry and Life Sciences (MicroTAS 2013), 27-31 October, Freiburg, Germany, pp. 128-130. (2013)

2. N.E. Steidle, M. Schneider, R. Ahrens, M. Worgull and A.E. Guber. *Fabrication of Polymeric Microfluidic Devices with Tunable Wetting Behavior for Biomedical Applications*, Proceedings of the 35th Annual International Conference of the IEEE Engineering in Medicine and Biology Society Conference (EMBC), 3. - 7. July 2013, Osaka, Japan, pp. 6659-6662. (2013)

3. N.E. Steidle, A. Lepple, M. Schneider, M. Heilig, R. Ahrens, M. Worgull and A.E. Guber. *Fabrication of Polymeric Microfluidic Devices by Microthermoforming for BioMEMS Applications*, Proceedings of the Polymer Processing Society 28th Annual Meeting, PPS-28, December 11-15, Pattaya, Thailand. (2012)

4. N.E. Steidle, S.M. Schillo, T. Fuchs, M. Schneider, R. Ahrens, M. Worgull, A. Nesterov-Mueller and A.E. Guber. *Fabrication of Micro- and Nanostructured Three-Dimensional Microchannels, to be submitted.* (2014)

5. N.E. Steidle, T. Hahn, M. Schneider, R. Ahrens, M. Worgull and A.E. Guber. *3-Dimensional Protein Immobilization on Micro- and Nanostructured Polymeric Surfaces, to be submitted.* (2014)

A.3. Conference Contributions

1. N.E. Steidle, T. Hahn, C. Bader, M. Schneider, R. Ahrens, M. Worgull and A.E. Guber. *Micro- and nanostructured microfluidic chip for specific protein immobilization*, Proceedings of the 17th International Conference on Miniaturized Systems for Chemistry and Life Sciences (MicroTAS 2013), 27-31 October, Freiburg, Germany, 2013. (*Poster Presentation*)

2. N.E. Steidle, M. Schneider, R. Ahrens, M. Worgull and A.E. Guber. *Fabrication of Polymeric Microfluidic Devices with Tunable Wetting Behavior for Biomedical Applications*, 35th Annual International Conference of the IEEE Engineering in Medicine and Biology Society Conference (EMBC), 3. - 7. July 2013, Osaka, Japan, 2013. (*Oral Presentation*)

3. N.E. Steidle, M. Schneider, R. Ahrens, M. Worgull, A.E. Guber. *Fabrication of Polymeric Microfluidic Devices for BioMEMS Applications*, 10th International Workshop on High Aspect Ratio Micro and Nano System Technology (HARMNST), 21-24 April, Berlin Germany, 2013. (*Poster Presentation*)

4. N.E. Steidle, A. Lepple, M. Schneider, M. Heilig, R. Ahrens, M. Worgull and A.E. Guber. *Fabrication of Polymeric Microfluidic Devices by Microthermoforming for BioMEMS Applications*, Polymer

Processing Society 28th Annual Meeting, PPS-28, December 11-15, Pattaya, Thailand, 2012. (*Oral Presentation*)

A.4. Seminar Talks at other Institutes

1. *Fabrication of Polymeric Microfluidic Devices with Micro- and Nanostructures for Biomedical Applications*, Group of E. Delamarche, IBM Research Zurich, Rüschlikon, Switzerland, September 26, 2013

2. *Fabrication of Polymeric Microfluidic Devices with Micro- and Nanostructures for Biomedical Applications*, Group of Prof. J. Brugger, Microsystems Laboratory (LMIS1), École Polytechnique Fédérale de Lausanne (EPFL), Lausanne, Switzerland, September 24, 2013

3. *Fabrication of Micro- and Nanostructured Polymeric Microfluidic Devices for Biomedical Applications*, Group of Prof. P. Dittrich, Bioanalytics Group, Eidgenössische Technische Hochschule (ETH) Zürich, Zurich, Switzerland, July 26, 2013

4. *Fabrication of Polymeric Microfluidic Devices with Tunable Wetting Behavior for Biomedical Applications*, Group of Prof. H. Yokoi, Institute of Industrial Science, University of Tokyo, Tokyo, Japan, July 12, 2013

List of Figures

2.1 Schematic view of the different domains of a protein. . . 7
2.2 Schematic depiction of the Contact Angle Hysteresis. . . 11
2.3 Schematic view of the Young state. 12
2.4 Schematic view of the a) Wenzel state and b) Cassie-Baxter state. 12
2.5 Dependency of the contact angle on the height of a pillar with a diameter of 15 µm.[40] 16
2.6 Influence of eccentricity on the dynamic contact angle and the contact angle hysteresis.[41] 17
2.7 Calculations of the contact angle after the Cassie-Baxter equation for PSU and COC. 19
2.8 SEM micrographs of the fabricated design layout. 20

3.1 Three-step fabrication process. 23
3.2 Schematic view of the hot embossing setup. 28
3.3 Schematic of the hot embossing process 30
3.4 Molding windows for amorphous and semicrystalline polymers.[68] 31
3.5 SEM micrograph of a hot embossed foil and the corresponding mold insert. 33
3.6 SEM micrograph of a double sided hot embossed foil. . . 34
3.7 Schematic view of the hot pulling demolding step. 35
3.8 SEM micrograph of hot pulled micro pillars with a top diameter of 9 µm and a height of 85 µm. 36

3.9 SEM micrographs comparing the results of different molding parameters with the same mold insert and material . . 36
3.10 SEM micrograph of a micropillar after direct laser writing with and without an anti-reflective layer. 38
3.11 Schematic view of the microthermoforming process. . . . 40
3.12 SEM micrograph of a thermoformed channel with microstructures on its surface. 41
3.13 Three dimensional model of the thermoformbonding process. 43
3.14 Schematic view of the twin-sheet-forming process. 44
3.15 Schematic view of the laser welding process. 47
3.16 Simplified view of the injection molding setup. 49

4.1 Contact angle measurement setup. 52
4.2 Results of dynamic contact angle measurements of PMMA, PSU, PC and COC with the same surface structure. 54
4.3 Results of static contact angle measurements for COC in dependency of pitch and diameter. 55
4.4 Velocity profile in a channel with a fluid in a) laminar flow and b) turbulent flow. 57
4.5 Schematic view of the no-slip, partial-slip and slip condition and the corresponding velocities. 61
4.6 Setup of micro astigmatism particle tracking velocimetry (μAPTV) measurements. 62
4.7 Results of μAPTV measurements. 63
4.8 Nikuradse diagram calculated from the μAPTV results. . 65
4.9 SEM micrographs of a) a tube after removing the residual layer with b) microstructures on the inside and c) nanostructures on the outside.[90] 67
4.10 Schematic view of the hot cutting mechanism. 68

4.11 Photography of a Micropipette with nanostructures on the inside. 69
4.12 Fluid in the Cassie-Baxter state and Wenzel state and apparent height of the channel. 71

5.1 Schematic view of the protein adsorption experiments. . . 77
5.2 SEM micrograph and fluorescence image with corresponding fluorescence intensity profile for one micro pillar. . . 78
5.3 SEM micrograph of a pillar with a diameter of 20 µm and fluorescence images taken with a laser scanning microscope. 80
5.4 Photography, SEM micrographs and fluorescence images of nanometer structures. 81
5.5 Results of BSA adsorption experiments on hot pulled surfaces. 82
5.6 Results of streptavidin adsorption experiments on hot pulled surfaces. 83
5.7 Comparison of Adsorption and Desorption of BSA on PSU and COC 84
5.8 Fluorescence image after a) adsorption and b) desorption of BSA on PSU on Field 3. 84
5.9 Comparison of fluorescence intensities of adsorbed BSA on COC and PSU 85
5.10 Preliminary experiment to examine functionality of adsorbed proteins. 89
5.11 Experimental setup for the detection of c-reactive protein. 90
5.12 Fluorescence images and intensity profiles a) before normalizing and b) after normalizing it to the background image. 91
5.13 Results of pre-experiments. 93
5.14 Results of sandwich assays for the detection of CRP in PBS. 94
5.15 Results of CRP in human serum 95

5.16 Portable read-out device for the Lab-on-a-Chip system developed by Bürkert Fluid Control Systems.[111] 97

6.1 Layout of different samples for cell experiments. 105
6.2 MDCK and C2C12 cell growth on a COC foil and a standard PS well plate after 24 and 96 hours. 105
6.3 C2C12 cell growth on unstructured and structured surfaces. 106

List of Tables

2.1 Classification of surfaces by their contact angle Θ_0. . . . 10

2.2 Advancing and receding contact angles (CA) of COC and PSU 18

3.1 Properties of the utilized polymers.[57] 26

3.2 Used parameters for drying polymers in a vacuum oven. . 30

3.3 List of hot embossing parameters with T_g being the glass transition temperature. 33

3.4 List of microthermoforming parameters. 41

4.1 Summary of utilized structures and channel dimensions with H being the Height, W being the Width of the channel, p being the pitch, d the diameter and h being the height of the structures. 62

4.2 Mean velocity, Reynolds number and Darcy friction factor calculated from the results of the µAPTV measurements. 64

4.3 Results of dynamic contact angle measurements. 65

5.1 Geometric properties (Dieamter (D), Pitch (P), Height (H), Elements per EC (EEC) and Circumference in EC (CEC)) of the used nanostructured foil. With the size of an elementary cell (EC) of 6 µm x 6 µm. 91

6.1 Geometrical properties of the used polymer foils for cell experiments. 104

Bibliography

[1] R. P. Feynman. There is plenty of room at the bottom. *Annual meeting of the American Physical Society at Caltech*, 1959.

[2] A. Heinrich, C. Lutz, S. Baumann, and I. Rau. A boy and his atom. *http://www.research.ibm.com*, 2013.

[3] W. Barthlott and C. Neinhuis. Purity of the sacred lotus, or escape from contamination in biological surfaces. *Planta*, 202(1):1 – 8, 1997.

[4] A. R. Parker and C. R. Lawrence. Water capture by a desert beetle. *Nature*, 414:33 – 34, 2001.

[5] D. W. Bechert, G. Hoppe, and W.-E. Reif. On the drag reduction of the shark skin. In *AIAA Shear Flow Control Conference*, 1985.

[6] P. Vukusic and J. R. Sambles. Photonic structures in biology. *Nature*, 424:852 – 855, 2003.

[7] A. E. Guber. Potential of microsystems in medicine. *Minimally Invasive Therapy*, 4:267 – 275, 1995.

[8] E. Wintermantel and S.-W. Ha. *Medizintechnik Life Science Engineering*. Springer Verlag, 5th edition, 2009.

[9] P. S. Dittrich, K. Tachikawa, and A. Manz. Micro total analysis systems. Latest advancements and trends. *Analytical Chemistry*, 78:3887 – 3907, 2006.

[10] J. El-Ali, P. K. Sorger, and K. F. Jensen. Cells on chips. *Nature*, 442:403 – 411, 2006.

[11] S. Nagrath, L. V. Sequist, S. Maheswaran, D. W. Bell, D. Irimia, L. Ulkus, M. R. Smith, E. L. Kwak, S. Digumarthy, A. Muzikansky, P. Ryan, U. J. Balis, R. G. Tompkins, D. A. Haber, and M. Toner. Isolation of rare circulating tumour cells in cancer patients by microchip technology. *Nature*, 450:1235 – 1239, 2007.

[12] P. S. Dittrich and A. Manz. Lab-on-a-Chip: microfluidics in drug discovery. *Nature*, 5:210 – 218, 2006.

[13] A. W. Martinez, S. T. Phillips, and G. M. Whitesides. Three-dimensional microfluidic devices fabricated in layered paper and tape. *Proceedings of the National Academy of Sciences of the United States of America*, 105:19606 – 19611, 2008.

[14] D. L. Nelson and M. Cox. *Lehninger Principles of Biochemistry*. Freeman, 6th [international ed.] edition, 2013.

[15] E. Sackmann and R. Merkel. *Lehrbuch der Biophysik*. Wiley-VCH Verlag, 2010.

[16] J. D. Andrade and V. Hlady. Protein adsorption and materials biocompatibility: A tutorial review and suggested hypotheses. In *Biopolymers/Non-Exclusion HPLC*, Advances in Polymer Science No. 79. Springer Verlag, 1986.

[17] J. Israelachvili. *Intermolecular and Surface Forces*. Academic Press Inc., 2nd edition, 1992.

[18] K. Nakanishi, T. Sakiyama, and K. Imamura. On the adsorption of proteins on solid surfaces, a common but very complicated phenomenon. *Journal of Bioscience and Bioengineering*, 91 (3):233 – 244, 2001.

[19] H.-J. Butt, K. Graf, and M. Kappl. *Physics and Chemistry of Interfaces*. Wiley-VCH Verlag, 2nd edition, 2006.

[20] W. Norde and J. Lyklema. Why proteins prefer interfaces. *Journal of Biomaterials Science, Polymer Edition*, 2 (3):183 – 202, 1991.

[21] M. Rabe, D. Verdes, and S. Seeger. Understanding protein adsorption phenomena at solid surfaces. *Advances in Colloid and Interface Science*, 162:87 – 106, 2011.

[22] K. Koch and W. Barthlott. Superhydrophobic and superhydrophilic plant surfaces: an inspiration for biomimetic materials. *Philosophical Transactions of the Royal Society A*, 367:1487 – 1509, 2009.

[23] T. Young. An essay on the cohesion of fluids. *Philosophical Transactions of the Royal Society of London*, 95:65 – 87, 1805.

[24] R. L. Wenzel. Resistance of solid surfaces to wetting by water. *Industrial and Engineering Chemistry*, 28 (8):987 – 994, 1936.

[25] A. B. D. Cassie and A. Baxter. Wettability of porous surfaces. *Transactions of the Faraday Society*, 40 (0):546 – 551, 1944.

[26] D. Quéré. Wetting and roughness. *Annual Review of Materials Research*, 38:71 – 99, 2008.

[27] E. Ostuni, C. S. Chen, D. E. Ingber, and G. M. Whitesides. Selective deposition of proteins and cells in arrays of microwells. *Langmuir*, 17:2828 – 2834, 2001.

[28] A. Bernard, J. P. Renault, B. Michel, H. R. Bosshard, and E. Delamarche. Microcontact printing of proteins. *Advanced Materials*, 12:1067 – 1070, 2000.

[29] E. Ueda, F. L. Geyer, V. Nedashkivska, and P. A. Levkin. Droplet microarrays: facile formation of arrays of microdroplets and hydrogel

micropads for cell screening applications. *Lab on a Chip*, 12:5218 – 5224, 2012.

[30] E. Kim, Y. Xia, and G. M. Whitesides. Polymer microstructures formed by moulding in capillaries. *Nature*, 376:581 – 584, 1995.

[31] H.-M. Song and C.-S. Lee. Simple fabrication of functionalized surface with polyethylene glycol microstructure and glycidyl methacrylate moiety for the selective immobilization of proteins and cells. *Korean Journal of Chemical Engineering*, 25 (6):1467 – 1472, 2008.

[32] K. Y. Suh, J. Seong, A. Khademhosseini, P. E. Laibinis, and R.T Langer. A simple soft lithographic route for fabrication of poly(ethylen glycol) microstructures for protein and cell patterning. *Biomaterials*, 25:557 – 563, 2004.

[33] M. A. Holden and P. S. Cramer. Light activated patterning of dye-labeled molecules on surfaces. *Journal of the American Chemical Society*, 125:8074 – 8075, 2003.

[34] A. Waldbaur, B. Waterkotte, K. Schmitz, and B. E. Rapp. Maskless projection lithography for the fast and flexible generation of grayscale protein patterns. *small*, 8 (10):1570 – 1578, 2012.

[35] A. S. Blawas and W. M. Reichert. Protein patterning. *Biomaterials*, 19, Issues 7-9:595 – 609, 1998.

[36] F. Rusmini, Z. Zhong, and J. Feijen. Protein immobilization strategies for protein biochips. *Biomacromolecules*, 8:1775 – 1789, 2007.

[37] L. S. Wong, F. Khan, and J. Micklefield. Selective covalent protein immobilization: Strategies and applications. *Chemical Reviews*, 109:4025 – 4063, 2009.

[38] N. J. Shirtcliffe, S. Aqil, C. Evanc, G. McHale, M. I. Newton, C. C. Perry, and P. Roach. The use of high aspect ratio photoresist (SU-8) for super-hydrophobic pattern prototyping. *Journal of Micromechanics and Microengineering*, 14:1384 – 1389, 2004.

[39] N. A. Patankar. On wettability of hydrophobic contact angles on rough surfaces. *Langmuir*, 19:1249 – 1253, 2003.

[40] N. J. Shirtcliffe, G. McHale, S. Atherton, and M. I. Newton. An introduction to superhydrophobicity. *Advances in Colloid and Interface Science*, 161:124 – 138, 2010.

[41] N. Kashaninejad, W. K. Chan, and N. T. Nguyen. Eccentricity effect of micropatterned surface on contact angle. *Langmuir*, 28 (10):4793 – 4799, 2012.

[42] D. Öner and T. J. McCarthy. Ultrahydrophobic surfaces. effects of topography length scales on wettability. *Langmuir*, 16:7777 – 7782, 2000.

[43] N. E. Steidle, M. Schneider, R. Ahrens, M. Worgull, and A.E. Guber. Fabrication of polymeric microfluidic devices with tunable wetting behavior for biomedical applications. In *Proceedings of the 35th Annual International Conference of the IEEE Engineering in Medicine and Biology Society Conference (EMBC), 3. - 7. July 2013, Osaka, Japan*, 2013.

[44] N. E. Steidle and T. Hahn. *Nanostrukturen/Bioreaktionen*. Patent Application: DE 10 2013 111 759, 2013.

[45] A. Albers. *Maschinenkonstruktionslehre I-III*. Karlsruher Institut für Technologie, 2005.

[46] D. C. Duffy, J. C. McDonald, J. A. Schueller, and G. M. Whitesides. Rapid prototyping of microfluidic systems in

poly(dimethylsiloxane). *Analytical Chemistry*, 79 (23):4974 – 4984, 1998.

[47] M. A. Eddings, M. A. Johnson, and B. K. Gale. Determining the optimal PDMS-PDMS bonding technique for microflluidic devices. *Journal of Micromechanics and Microengineering*, 18:1 – 4, 2008.

[48] A. E. Guber. *Personal Information from Prof. A. E. Guber*. 2013.

[49] A. Waldbaur, H. Rapp, K. Länge, and B. E. Rapp. Let there be chip - towards rapid prototyping of microfluidic devices: one-step manufacturing processes. *Analytical Methods*, 3:2681 – 2716, 2011.

[50] T. D. Boone, Z. H. Fan, H. H. Hooper, A. J. Ricco, H. Tan, and S. J. Williams. Plastic advances microfluidic devices. *Analytical Chemistry*, 74 (3):78 A – 86 A, 2002.

[51] J. Heneka, M. Guttmann, K. Plewa, J. Mohr, T. Hanemann, and V. Saile. LIGA2.x process for mass proproduct of single polymeric LIGA micro parts. *Microsystem Technologies*, pages 1 – 6, 2013.

[52] B. Farshchian, S. Park, J. Choi, A. Amirsadeghi, J. Lee, and S. Park. 3D nanomolding for lab-on-a -chip applications. *Lab on a Chip*, 12:4764 – 4771, 2012.

[53] H. Lim, J. Ryu, G. Kim, K.-B. Choi, S. Lee, and J. Lee. Nanoimprint lithographiy with a focused laser beam for the fabrication of nanopatterned microchannel molds. *Lab on a Chip*, 13:3188 – 3191, 2013.

[54] P. Eyerer, T. Hirth, and P. Elsner. *Polymer Engineering*. Springer Verlag, 2008.

[55] R. J. Young and P. A. Lovell. *Introduction to Polymers*. CRC Press, Taylor and Francis Group, LLC, 2011.

[56] D. Walton and P. Lorimer. *Polymers*. Oxfort Chemistry Primers No. 85. Oxford University Press, 2005.

[57] H. Domininghaus, P. Elsner, P. Eyerer, and T. Hirth. *Kunststoffe*. Springer Verlag, 7th edition, 2008.

[58] Lipp-Terler. LITE U (PSU) datasheet. *LITE GmbH*, www.lipp-terler.com, 2013.

[59] W. M. Haynes, D. R. Lide, and T. J. Bruno. *CRC Handbook of Chemistry and Physics*. CRC Press, Taylor and Francis Group, LLC, 93rd edition, 2012.

[60] Topas. COC datasheet. *TOPAS Advanced Polymers*, www.topas.com, 2006.

[61] BASF. PSU datasheet. *BASF Plastics*, www.plasticsportal.com, 2010.

[62] M. J. Vasile, C. R. Friedrich, B. Kikkeri, and R. McElhannon. Micrometer-scale machining: tool fabrication and initial results. *Precision Engineering*, 19:180 – 186, 1996.

[63] N. E. Steidle, N. Takama, and B. J. Kim. Fast fabrication of micro tools with WEDG in deionized water. In *Proceedings of the 10th Korean MEMS Conference, 3 - 5 April, 2008, Jeju Island, Kore, pp. 105 - 106*, 2008.

[64] M. Guttmann, J. Schulz, and V. Saile. Lithographic fabrication of mold inserts. In *Microengineering of Metals and Ceramics: Part I: Design, Tooling and Injection Molding*, Advanced Micro and Nanosystems Volume 3. WILEY-VCH Verlag GmbH und Co. KGaA, 2005.

[65] J. Fischer and M. Wegener. Three-dimensional direct laser writing inspired by sitimulated-emission-depletion microscopy. *Optical Materials Express*, 614, 2011.

[66] M. Röhrig, M. Thiel, M. Worgull, and H. Hölscher. 3D direct laser writing of nano- and microstructured hierarchical gecko-mimicking surfaces. *Small*, 8 (19):3009 – 3015, 2012.

[67] M. Heckele, W. Bacher, and K. D. Mueller. Hot embossing - the molding technique for plastic microstructures. *Microsystem Tecnologies*, 4:122 – 124, 1998.

[68] M. Worgull. *Hot Embossing: Theory and Technology of Microreplication*. Micro & Nano Technologies. William Andrew, Oxford, 2009.

[69] P. C. Vella, S. S. Dimov, A. Kolew, E. Minev, K. Popov, F. Lacan, C. Griffiths, H. Hirshy, and S. Scholz. Bulk metallic glass based tool-making process chain for micro- and nano-replication. In *Proceedings of the 9th International Conference on Multi-Material Micro Manufacture (4M), 9 - 11 October, Vienna, Austria*, 2012.

[70] G. Kumar, H. X. Tang, and J. Schroers. Nanomoulding with amorphous metals. *Nature*, 457:868 – 873, 2009.

[71] M. Worgull, M. Schneider, M. Röhrig, T. Meier, M. Heilig, A. Kolew, K. Feit, H. Hölscher, and J. Leuthold. Hot embossing and thermoforming of biodegradable three-dimensional wood structures. *RSC Advances*, 3:20060 – 20064, 2013.

[72] A. Frick and C. Stern. *DSC-Prüfung in der Anwendung*. Hanser Verlag, 2nd edition, 2013.

[73] R. Truckenmueller, S. Giselbrecht, N. Rivron, E. Gottwald, V. Saile, A. van den Berg, M. Wessling, and C. van Blitterswijk. Thermo-

forming of film-based biomedical microdevices. *Advanced Materials*, 23:1311 – 1329, 2011.

[74] M. Heilig, M. Schneider, H. Dinglreiter, and M. Worgull. Technology of microthermoforming of complex three-dimensional parts with multiscale features. *Microsystem Technologies*, 17:593 – 600, 2011.

[75] J. L. Throne and J. Beine. *Thermoformen: Werkstoffe - Verfahren - Anwendungen*. Carl Hanser Verlag München Wien, 1999.

[76] M. J. Madou. *Fundamentals of Microfabrication and Nanotechnology Volume III - From MEMS to Bio-MEMS and Bio-NEMS*. CRC Press, Taylor and Francis Group, LLC, 3rd edition, 2012.

[77] C.-W. Tsao and D. L. DeVoe. Bonding of thermoplastic polymer microfluidics. *Microfluidics and Nanofluidics*, 6:1 – 16, 2009.

[78] X Han and H. Yokoi. Visualization analysis of the filling behavior of melt into microscale v-grooves during the filling stage of injection molding. *Polymer Engineering & Science*, 46 (11):1590 – 1597, 2006.

[79] M. R. Kamal, A. I. Isayev, and S.-J. Liu. *Injection Molding: Technology and Fundamentals*. Hanser Verlag, 2009.

[80] F. Johannaber and W. Michaeli. *Handbuch Spritzgießen*. Carl Hanser Verlag München, 2nd edition, 2004.

[81] N. E. Steidle, S. M. Schillo, T. Fuchs, M. Schneider, S. Huang, R. Ahrens, M. Worgull, A. Nesterov-Mueller, and A. E. Guber. Fabrication of micro- and nanostructured three-dimensional microchannels. *to be submitted*, 2014.

[82] J. Spurk and N. Aksel. *Fluid Mechanics*. Springer Verlag, 2008.

[83] L. Böswirth. *Technische Strömungslehre*. Vieweg + Teubner Verlag, 8th edition, 2010.

[84] W. Bohl and E. Elmendorf. *Technische Strömungslehre*. Vogel Fachbuch Kamprath-Reihe, 2008.

[85] W. Kast and H. Nirschl. Druckverlust in einphasigen Strömungen. In *VDI-Wärmeatlas*, VDI-Buch. Springer Verlag, 2013.

[86] G. Hetsroni, A. Mosyak, E. Pogrebnyak, and L. P. Yarin. Fluid flow in micro-channels. *International Journal of Heat and Mass Transfer*, 48:1982 – 1998, 2005.

[87] C. Tropea, A. L. Yarin, and J. F. Foss. *Springer Handbook of Experimental Fluid Mechanics*. Springer Verlag, 2007.

[88] C. Cierpka and C. J. Kähler. Particle imaging techniques for volumetric three-component (3D3C) velocity measurements in microfluidics. *Journal of Visualization*, 15 (1):1 – 31, 2012.

[89] F. Falkensteiner, A. Steininger, and G. Müller. Katheterassoziierte Komplikationen und Liegedauer peripherer Venenverweilkanülen - Eine Literaturübersicht. *pro care*, 16 (5):11 – 16, 2011.

[90] N. E. Steidle, A. Lepple, M. Schneider, M. Heilig, R. Ahrens, M. Worgull, and A. E. Guber. Fabrication of polymeric microfluidic devices by microthermoforming for BioMEMS applications. In *Proceedings of the Polymer Processing Society 28th Annual Meeting, PPS-28, December 11-15, Pattaya, Thailand*, 2012.

[91] M. L. W. Knetsch and L. H. Koole. New strategies in the development of antimicrobial coatings: The example of increasing usage of silver and silver nanoparticles. *Polymers*, 3:340 – 366, 2011.

[92] D. L. Elbert and J. A. Hubbel. Surface treatments of polymers for biocompatibility. *Annual Review of Material Science*, 26:365 – 394, 1996.

[93] P. Harder, M. Grunze, R. Dahing, G. M. Whitesides, and P. E. Laibinis. Molecular conformation in oligo(ethylene glycol)-terminated self-assembled monolayers on gold and silver surfaces determines their ability to resist protein adsorption. *Journal of Physical Chemistry B*, 102 (2):426 – 436, 1998.

[94] F. Kessler, D. Steffens, G. A. Lando, P. Pranke, and D. E. Weibel. Wettability and cell spreading enhancement in poly(sulfone) and polyurethane surfaces by UV-assisted treatment for tissue engineering purposes. *Tissue Engineering and Regenerative Medicine*, 11 (1):22 – 31, 2014.

[95] N. E. Steidle, T. Hahn, C. Bader, M. Schneider, R. Ahrens, M. Worgull, and A. E. Guber. Micro- and nanostructured microfluidic chip for specific protein immobilization. In *Proceedings of the 17th International Conference on Miniaturized Systems for Chemistry and Life Sciences (MicroTAS 2013), 27 - 31 October, Freiburg, Germany, pp. 128-130*, 2013.

[96] K. Länge. *Personal Information from Dr. Kerstin Länge*. 2013.

[97] F. W. D. Rost. *Fluorescence microscopy*, volume I. Cambridge University Press, 1992.

[98] M. Hoppert. *Microscopic Techniques in Biotechnology*. Wiley-VCH Verlag, 2003.

[99] G. T. Hermanson. *Bioconjugate Techniques*. Academic Press Inc., 2nd edition, 2008.

[100] T. Grossmann, M. Hauser, T. Beck, C. Gohn-Kreuz, M. Karl, C. Vannahme, and T. Mappes. High-Q conical polymeric microcavities. *Applied Physics Letters*, 96:013303, 2010.

[101] W. Zhang, N. Ganesh, I. D. Block, and B. T. Cunningham. High sensitivity photonic crystal biosensor incorporating nanorod structures for enhanced surface area. *Sensors and Actuators, B: Chemical*, 131:279 – 284, 2008.

[102] life technologies. *The Molecular Probes Handbook*. life technologies, 11th edition, 2010.

[103] Sigma-Aldrich. *Product Information: Albumin From Bovine Serum (BSA)*. http://www.sigmaaldrich.com, 2014.

[104] L.-C. Sang, A. Vinu, and M.-O. Coppens. General description of the adsorption of proteins at their isoelectric point in nanoporous materials. *Langmuir*, 27:13828 – 13837, 2011.

[105] F. J. Gruhl, B. E. Rapp, and K. Länge. Biosensors for diagnostic applications. In *Molecular Diagnostics*, Advances in Biochemical Engineering/Biotechnologie, No. 133, pages 115 – 148. Springer Verlag, 2013.

[106] P. Bertoncello and R. J. Forster. Nanostructured materials for electrochemiluminescence (ECL)-based detection methods: recent advances and future perspectives. *Biosensors and Bioelectronics*, 24:3191 – 3200, 2009.

[107] X. Fan, I. M. White, S. I. Shopova, H. Zhu, J. D. Suter, and Y. Sun. Sensitive optical biosensors for unlabeled targets: A review. *Analytica Chimica Acta*, 620:8 – 26, 2008.

[108] B. Liedberg, C. Nylander, and I. Lundstrom. Surface plasmon resonance for gas detection and biosensing. *Sensors and Actuators*, 4:299 – 304, 1983.

[109] A. Abbas, M. J. Linman, and Q. Cheng. New trends in instrumental design for surface plasmon resonance-base biosensors. *Biosensors and Bioelectronics*, 26 (5):1815 – 1824, 2011.

[110] C. Albrecht, N. Kaeppel, and G. Gauglitz. Two immunoassay formats for fully automated CRP detection in human serum. *Analytical and Bioanalytical Chemistry*, 391:1845 – 1852, 2008.

[111] T. Hahn. *Portabler Mikrofluidik kPrototyp für ultrasensitive Fluoreszenzauswertung*. MicroTec Südwest, MSTBW Clusterconference 2014, 5 - 6 May, 2014, Freiburg, Germany, 2014.

[112] J. R. Rettig and A. Folch. Large-scale single-cell trapping and imaging using microwell arrays. *Analytical Chemistry*, 77:5628 – 5634, 2005.

[113] Y. Kuang, I. Biran, and D. R. Walt. Simultaneously monitoring gene expression kinetics and genetic noise in single cell by optical well arrays. *Analytical Chemistry*, 76:6282 – 6286, 2004.

[114] D. DiCarlo, L. Y. Wu, and L. P. Lee. Dynamic single cell culture array. *Lab on a Chip*, 6:1445 – 1449, 2006.

[115] A. R. Wheeler, W. R. Throndset, R. J. Whelan, A. M. Leach, R. N. Zare, Y. H. Liao, K. Farrell, I. D. Manger, and A. Daridon. Microfluidic device for single-cell analysis. *Analytical Chemistry*, 75:3581 – 3586, 2003.

[116] U. Seger, S. Gawad, R. Johann, A. Bertsch, and P. Renaud. Cell immersion and cell dipping in microfluidic devices. *Lab on a Chip*, 4:148 – 151, 2004.

[117] M. Suzuki, T. Yasukawa, H. Shiku, and T. Matsue. Analysis dielectrophoretic patterning with different cell types. *Biosensors and Bioelectronics*, 24:1043 – 1047, 2008.

[118] E. Martinez, E. Engel, J. A. Planell, and J. Samitier. Effects of artificial micro- and nano-structured surfaces on cell behaviour. *Annals of Anatomy-Anatomischer Anzeiger*, 191 (1):126 – 135, 2009.

[119] S.-H. Yoon, Y. K. Kim, E. D. Han, Y.-H. Seo, B. H. Kime, and M. R. K. Mofrad. Passive control of cell locomotion using micropatterns: the effect of micropattern geometry on the migratory behavior of adherent cells. *Lab on a Chip*, 12:2391 – 2402, 2012.

[120] F. Klein, T. Striebel, J. Fischer, Z. Jiang, C. M. Fran, G. von Freymann, M. Wegener, and M. Bastmeyer. Elastic fully three-dimensional microstructure scaffolds for cell force measurements. *Advanced Materials*, 22:868 – 871, 2010.

[121] F. Klein, B. Richter, T. Striebel, C. M. Franz, G. von Freymann, M. Wegener, and M. Bastmeyer. Two-component polymer scaffolds for controlled three-dimensional cell culture. *Advanced Materials*, 23:1341 – 1345, 2011.

[122] J. L. Tan, J. Tien, D. M. Pirone, D. S. Gray, K. Bhadriraju, and C. S. Chen. Cells lying on a bed of microneedles: An approach to isolate mechanical force. *Proceedings of the National Academy of Sciences of the United States of America*, 100 (4):1484 – 1489, 2003.

[123] J. Fu, Y.-K. Wang, M. T. Yan, R. A. Desai, X. Yu, Z. Liu, and S. C. Chen. Mechanical regulation of cell function with geometrically modulated elastomeric substrates. *Nature Methods*, 7 (9):733 – 736, 2010.

[124] B. Alberts, D. Bray, K. Hopkin, A. Johnson, J. Lewis, M. Raff, K. Roberts, and P. Walter. *Essential Cell Biology*. Garland Science, 2010.

[125] G. C. Karp. *Cell Biology*. John Wiley & Sons, 2010.

[126] R. I. Freshney. *Culture of Animal Cells*. Wiley-Blackwell, 6th edition, 2010.

[127] T. Lindl and G. Gstraunthaler. *Zell- und Gewebekultur*. Spektrum Akademischer Verlag, 6th edition, 2008.

[128] J. W. Haycock. 3d cell culture: A review of current approaches and techniques. In *3D Cell Culture*. Springer Verlag, 2011.

[129] J. Engel and M. Chiquet. An overview of extracellular matrix structure and function. In *The Extracellular Matrix: an Overview*. Springer Verlag, 2011.

[130] E. D. Hay. *Cell Biology of Extracellular Matrix*. Plenum Press, 2nd edition, 1991.

[131] J. Lee, M. J. Cuddihy, and N. A. Kotov. Three-dimensional cell culture matrices: State of the art. *Tissue Engineering: Part B*, 14 (1):61 – 86, 2008.

[132] P. L. Roberts. Sterilization. In *Animal Cell Culture*. Wiley-Blackwell, 2011.

[133] D. Yaffe and O. Saxel. Serial passaging and differentiation of myogenic cells isolated from dystrophic mouse muscle. *Nature*, 270:725 – 727, 1977.

[134] S. H. Madin and N. B. Darby Jr. Established kidney cell lines of normal adult bovine and ovine origin. *Experimental Biology and Medicine*, 122 (3):931 – 935, 1958.

[135] R. Pankov and K. M. Yamada. Fibronectin at a glance. *Journal of Cell Science*, 115:3861 – 3863, 2002.

[136] F. Kurth, K. Eyer, A. Franco-Obregón, and P. S. Dittrich. A new mechanobiological era: microfluidic pathways to apply and sense

forces at the cellular level. *Current Opinion in Chemical Biology*, 16:400 – 408, 2012.

[137] O. du Roure, A. Saez, A. Buguin, R. H. Austin, P. Chavrier, P. Silberzan, and B. Ladoux. Force mapping in epithelial cell migration. *Proceedings of the National Academy of Sciences of the United States of America*, 102 (39):2390 – 2395, 2005.

Schriften des Instituts für Mikrostrukturtechnik
am Karlsruher Institut für Technologie (KIT)

ISSN 1869-5183

Herausgeber: Institut für Mikrostrukturtechnik

Die Bände sind unter www.ksp.kit.edu als PDF frei verfügbar
oder als Druckausgabe zu bestellen.

Band 1 **Georg Obermaier**
Research-to-Business Beziehungen: Technologietransfer durch Kommunikation von Werten (Barrieren, Erfolgsfaktoren und Strategien). 2009
ISBN 978-3-86644-448-5

Band 2 **Thomas Grund**
Entwicklung von Kunststoff-Mikroventilen im Batch-Verfahren. 2010
ISBN 978-3-86644-496-6

Band 3 **Sven Schüle**
Modular adaptive mikrooptische Systeme in Kombination mit Mikroaktoren. 2010
ISBN 978-3-86644-529-1

Band 4 **Markus Simon**
Röntgenlinsen mit großer Apertur. 2010
ISBN 978-3-86644-530-7

Band 5 **K. Phillip Schierjott**
Miniaturisierte Kapillarelektrophorese zur kontinuierlichen Überwachung von Kationen und Anionen in Prozessströmen. 2010
ISBN 978-3-86644-523-9

Band 6 **Stephanie Kißling**
Chemische und elektrochemische Methoden zur Oberflächenbearbeitung von galvanogeformten Nickel-Mikrostrukturen. 2010
ISBN 978-3-86644-548-2

Schriften des Instituts für Mikrostrukturtechnik
am Karlsruher Institut für Technologie (KIT)

ISSN 1869-5183

Band 7 Friederike J. Gruhl
Oberflächenmodifikation von Surface Acoustic Wave (SAW) Biosensoren für biomedizinische Anwendungen. 2010
ISBN 978-3-86644-543-7

Band 8 Laura Zimmermann
Dreidimensional nanostrukturierte und superhydrophobe mikrofluidische Systeme zur Tröpfchengenerierung und -handhabung. 2011
ISBN 978-3-86644-634-2

Band 9 Martina Reinhardt
Funktionalisierte, polymere Mikrostrukturen für die dreidimensionale Zellkultur. 2011
ISBN 978-3-86644-616-8

Band 10 Mauno Schelb
Integrierte Sensoren mit photonischen Kristallen auf Polymerbasis. 2012
ISBN 978-3-86644-813-1

Band 11 Daniel Auernhammer
Integrierte Lagesensorik für ein adaptives mikrooptisches Ablenksystem. 2012
ISBN 978-3-86644-829-2

Band 12 Nils Z. Danckwardt
Pumpfreier Magnetpartikeltransport in einem Mikroreaktionssystem: Konzeption, Simulation und Machbarkeitsnachweis. 2012
ISBN 978-3-86644-846-9

Band 13 Alexander Kolew
Heißprägen von Verbundfolien für mikrofluidische Anwendungen. 2012
ISBN 978-3-86644-888-9

Schriften des Instituts für Mikrostrukturtechnik
am Karlsruher Institut für Technologie (KIT)

ISSN 1869-5183

Band 14 Marko Brammer
Modulare Optoelektronische Mikrofluidische Backplane. 2012
ISBN 978-3-86644-920-6

Band 15 Christiane Neumann
Entwicklung einer Plattform zur individuellen Ansteuerung von Mikroventilen und Aktoren auf der Grundlage eines Phasenüberganges zum Einsatz in der Mikrofluidik. 2013
ISBN 978-3-86644-975-6

Band 16 Julian Hartbaum
Magnetisches Nanoaktorsystem. 2013
ISBN 978-3-86644-981-7

Band 17 Johannes Kenntner
Herstellung von Gitterstrukturen mit Aspektverhältnis 100 für die Phasenkontrastbildgebung in einem Talbot-Interferometer. 2013
ISBN 978-3-7315-0016-2

Band 18 Kristina Kreppenhofer
Modular Biomicrofluidics - Mikrofluidikchips im Baukastensystem für Anwendungen aus der Zellbiologie. 2013
ISBN 978-3-7315-0036-0

Band 19 Ansgar Waldbaur
Entwicklung eines maskenlosen Fotolithographiesystems zum Einsatz im Rapid Prototyping in der Mikrofluidik und zur gezielten Oberflächenfunktionalisierung. 2013
ISBN 978-3-7315-0119-0

Band 20 Christof Megnin
Formgedächtnis-Mikroventile für eine fluidische Plattform. 2013
ISBN 978-3-7315-0121-3

Schriften des Instituts für Mikrostrukturtechnik
am Karlsruher Institut für Technologie (KIT)

ISSN 1869-5183

Band 21 Srinivasa Reddy Yeduru
Development of Microactuators Based on
the Magnetic Shape Memory Effect. 2013
ISBN 978-3-7315-0125-1

Band 22 Michael Röhrig
Fabrication and Analysis of Bio-Inspired Smart Surfaces. 2014
ISBN 978-3-7315-0163-3

Band 23 Taleieh Rajabi
Entwicklung eines mikrofluidischen Zweikammer-
Chipsystems mit integrierter Sensorik für die Anwendung
in der Tumorforschung. 2014
ISBN 978-3-7315-0220-3

Band 24 Frieder Märkle
Laserbasierte Verfahren zur Herstellung hochdichter
Peptidarrays. 2014
ISBN 978-3-7315-0222-7

Band 25 Tobias Meier
Magnetoresistive and Thermoresistive Scanning
Probe Microscopy with Applications in Micro- and
Nanotechnology. 2014
ISBN 978-3-7315-0253-1

Band 26 Felix Marschall
Entwicklung eines Röntgenmikroskops für
Photonenenergien von 15 keV bis 30 keV. 2014
ISBN 978-3-7315-0263-0

Band 27 Leonardo Pires Carneiro
Development of an Electrochemical Biosensor Platform and a
Suitable Low-Impedance Surface Modification Strategy. 2014
ISBN 978-3-7315-0272-2

Schriften des Instituts für Mikrostrukturtechnik
am Karlsruher Institut für Technologie (KIT)

ISSN 1869-5183

Band 28 **Sebastian Mathias Schillo**
Prozessentwicklung für die Automatisierung der Herstellung und Anwendung von hochdichten Peptidmicroarrays. 2014
ISBN 978-3-7315-0274-6

Band 29 **Nicole E. Steidle**
Micro- and Nanostructured Microfluidic Devices for Localized Protein Immobilization and Other Biomedical Applications. 2014
ISBN 978-3-7315-0297-5